Careers in
Hairdressing
and
Beauty Therapy

Sixth Edition

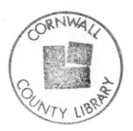

ALEXA STACE

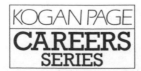

LIS 6/02

First published in 1980
Second edition 1983
Third edition 1985
Fourth edition 1988
Fifth edition 1990
Sixth edition 1993, revised and updated by Carol Woolley

Kogan Page Limited
120 Pentonville Road
London N1 9JN

© Kogan Page Ltd 1980, 1983, 1985, 1988, 1990, 1993

British Library Cataloguing in Publication Data

A CIP record for this book is available from the British Library.

ISBN 0-7494-1060-4

Typeset by DP Photosetting, Aylesbury, Bucks
Printed and bound in Great Britain by
Clays Ltd, St Ives plc

Introduction

Throughout the ages people have been interested in their personal appearance. Cosmetics were used by the ancient Egyptians, while the use of sauna baths, exercise and massage to improve physical fitness was well known to the Greeks and Romans.

Today, with the ever-increasing accent on youth, there is more interest than ever, particularly as the services of hairdressers, beauty firms, sauna establishments etc are within the reach of everyone, not just a privileged few. Cosmetic firms produce ranges to suit everyone's pocket, from the teenage products sold in chain stores such as Woolworth's to the exclusive French-made products, and staff are needed to market, sell and demonstrate these ranges. Beauty salons are now almost as familiar as hairdressers in the local high street and there, too, there is a demand for qualified staff.

At one time cosmetics were regarded very much as camouflage, to hide the ravages of time or disease. Now, with the increasingly scientific approach to beauty, research chemists spend their working lives perfecting creams and lotions that will prevent wrinkles and hold off the effects of ageing for as long as possible. The scientific approach has also meant an increasing use of electrical and electronic equipment in the treatment of face and body, and the beauty therapist must learn how to handle all this equipment with confidence.

This scientific approach is also seen in hairdressing. An increasing number of people are having their hair streaked, tinted, coloured or permed and the hairdresser must have a basic knowledge of chemistry to understand what is happening. All the main techniques are covered during training.

Another fairly recent development has been the realisation that health and beauty go hand in hand, leading to an upsurge of interest in keeping fit. The cult of youth, too, has meant that everyone wants to look slim and youthful, and so there has been a great increase in the numbers of health clubs, health farms, sauna baths etc. Dance and exercise help clients to become fit and slim through vigorous workouts – there are several different 'methods' to choose from, as well as yoga and self-defence. Many local authorities have now installed sauna and steam baths in their sports centres and all these establishments need trained staff to run them.

People with a training in massage – especially remedial massage – are especially in demand.

All jobs in hairdressing, beauty therapy, health and fitness involve supplying a personal service, so your appearance and manner towards other people will obviously be crucial. We have therefore included a chapter on how to apply for jobs (or apprenticeships) and how to behave at interviews, with a checklist of dos and don'ts to help you put your best foot forward. It's not good looks, but good manners and good grooming that will get you the job.

Part 1

Chapter 1

Hairdressing

Hairdressing is a very important aspect of the beauty world. Most women realise the importance of a good cut, and many go for 'extras' such as highlights or tints. Also, many older women have their hair washed and set professionally once a week, while more and more men too are having their hair 'styled' at a hairdresser's rather than simply cut at the barber's. Hairdressing, in fact, is big business.

Many establishments now, especially in the larger towns and cities, are unisex, with both male and female clients coming regularly to have their hair permed, coloured, tinted, washed and styled. The increasing accent for both sexes on healthy, youthful looks means that people want to disguise greying or thinning hair; they want out-of-condition hair treated, and they want to keep up with the changing fashions in hairstyles, whether long or short, straight or curly; here they will look to the hairdresser for advice.

All this means ever-increasing custom for the hairdresser, who has to be skilled in all the various techniques of perming, colouring, tinting, waving and setting. Perming, colouring and bleaching are used widely, and the hairdresser must take great care in handling the chemicals involved. It is often quite difficult to achieve the effect the client wants; all sorts of factors, such as the condition of the hair, its texture, and previous treatments, particularly bleaching, can affect the final result. In large salons there is often a special department where clients go for such treatments. The staff will have specialised in these particular techniques and will probably have attended a course organised by one of the manufacturers to learn more about the latest colouring and waving techniques.

In a smaller salon, of course, the qualified hairdresser will be expected to cope with whatever treatment the client requires. The smaller the salon, in fact, the more varied the work.

Most hairdressers are employed in high street salons up and down the country, but salons can also be found in hotels, clubs, department stores, airports and on large passenger liners. Some of the shipping companies require a knowledge of beauty culture as well as a hairdressing qualification.

Qualities Required

Hairdressing is very much a personal service, so it is essential to have a warm, friendly and sympathetic manner. You may be a brilliant artist with the scissors, but if you have a brusque, unfriendly manner your clients are unlikely to return. A hairdresser can soon gauge his or her success, in fact, by the number of regular clients acquired.

It helps if you have a calm, unflappable nature – tempers can run high in a busy, crowded salon – and the ability to talk easily to all kinds of people. You also have to be very patient, particularly when dealing with children who often object to having their hair cut and dislike sitting still for long periods.

Obviously you should be good at working with your hands, as well as being both observant and interested in other people. Good health is important – this is a tiring job and the hairdresser rarely sits down. On a busy day the popular stylist will find little time for lunch or coffee breaks – stamina is needed for this job. It helps too if you are of average height; very tall and very short people will find the constant bending and reaching exhausting.

Personal appearance is also important. The hairdresser, of either sex, should be well groomed and well turned out. The stylist whose own hair is a mess will not inspire confidence in a client. Hands should be clean and well kept, without bitten nails, and no one with dermatitis is advised to consider a career in hairdressing.

Training

There are five different ways of training:

1. A two-year placement on Youth Training (YT), offering on-the-job experience and off-the-job training. It is not unusual for YT trainees to be 'employed status' apprentices.
2. A two-, or occasionally three-year apprenticeship in a hairdressing salon, ideally with provision for attending day-release or evening classes at a Hairdressing Training Board/City and Guilds registered centre.

3. A two-year, full-time course at a further education college.
4. A private school course, usually lasting from six to nine months.
5. An Employment Training (shortly to be known as Training for Employment) programme.

The City and Guilds Institute, working jointly with the Hairdressing Training Board, is currently developing National Vocational Qualifications (NVQs) which are at the following levels:

(a) NVQ Level 1 is designed for use in schools, for people with Saturday jobs, or for those with special training needs. It includes assisting with reception duties, handling stock, ensuring a healthy and safe environment and liaising with clients.

(b) NVQ Level 2 is for those who wish to learn the basic skills to become competent hairdressers, such as receiving and checking out clients, diagnosing hair and scalp conditions, shampooing, cutting, setting, perming and colouring hair. A second award at Level 2 includes a competence in relaxing and straightening Afro-type hair.

(c) NVQ Level 3 is designed for the aspiring supervisor as it covers skills such as training, monitoring and stock control. It is also for those who wish to extend their technical skills in response to the latest developments.

(d) NVQ Level 4 is appropriate for salon managers and covers control, development and utilisation of resources, business planning and quality control.

NB In Scotland there is a comparable vocational qualification (SVQ) (see pp 63-4).

YT Trainees/Apprentices

Both YT and apprenticeships provide the opportunity to acquire practical experience right from the start. At the beginning, as a trainee or apprentice, you will be a general dogsbody, expected to fetch and carry for the stylists. You will have to shampoo clients, hand up pins and clips, make tea and coffee and keep the salon tidy. You will also have to look after the clients by fetching magazines, coffee etc, and hanging up coats.

Your training will start with being taught how to look after the equipment and materials in the salon - scissors, brushes, combs, electrical equipment etc. You will be shown the basic hairdressing operations - the correct way to brush and comb, how to shampoo, how to give a colour rinse and eventually how to cut hair. From the start, trainees and apprentices learn a lot by watching the experienced staff at work. Many of the larger salons set aside one evening a week for practice and instruction by the senior staff, and you would be well advised to get additional training at an HTB/C&G registered centre, leading to the qualifications described above.

As you gain experience, you are introduced to permanent waving and colouring and may be asked to attend one of the short courses arranged by the manufacturers. You may have the chance, under supervision, to wind perms and do colouring. It is important to understand the effects on the hair and the skin of the various chemicals used – it helps if you did some science or chemistry at school.

Full-time Courses
A large number of colleges run full-time courses leading either to their own award or to NVQs.

Private Hairdressing Schools
Private schools usually run short, intensive courses – six to nine months is the average. There are no particular educational qualifications, but a good general education is always preferred.

Fees tend to be high, so you should make careful enquiries about your future job prospects before committing yourself to a private course.

Some of the large firms owning a chain of salons run their own schools, and these will often help to place you after training. It is a good idea to ask your Jobcentre or local Careers Office for advice before registering with a particular school to ensure that the training offered will help in finding a job.

There are many excellent hairdressing schools but two of the top ones are:

1. Graham Webb International School of Hairdressing, 202–204 High Street, Eltham, London SE9 1BD. Courses vary from a 30-week intensive NVQ for beginners at £2,990, to refresher courses from £200 to £1,990, and an advanced course costing £230.
2. The world-renowned Vidal Sassoon School, based at 56–58 Davies Mews, London W1Y 1AS and other centres in London and Manchester, offers several courses from a one-week classic course at £325 to either a 16-week foundation course costing £3,500 or a 35-week beginners' diploma costing £6,500, both leading to the City and Guilds NVQ.

Wigmaking

For anyone interested in the art of wigmaking (which may be

covered in Hairdressing and Beauty Therapy courses) there are many other opportunities for the dedicated. Apart from working in a television studio or with wax models, film studios have a constant need for wigs, particularly for period films, as does the live stage. In the field of fashion too there is a demand for wigs for live mannequins and models, and for dressing dummies for shop window displays. Many members of the public wear wigs, either as a necessity (on medical grounds) or as a change purely for reasons of fashion. However, it is as well to point out that jobs connected with television, film studios and the theatre are much sought after, and the competition is therefore keen.

Madame Tussauds of London employs two wigmakers, although most wax heads have hair inserted strand by strand, a job requiring special additional training. No back-chat from clients and certainly a job with a difference! It goes without saying that such jobs are much coveted and applicants need to be fully trained in hairdressing and, ideally, have some art training as well.

Case Studies
Linda Franks is head stylist in a large West End salon in London.

The best advice I can give any youngster going into this business is to get a really good training. It is important to train in a top-class salon if you can possibly manage it. This salon, for example, is a marvellous place to do your training. The management take a lot of trouble with the trainees and we all try to help them all we can. It's a very busy salon and we have a varied clientèle, so they get a lot of different experience and that's important. We have a training session when they get put through their paces and we take it in turns to do demonstrations for them.

I enjoy the work enormously. You are always meeting new people and they are usually pretty interesting, with fairly exciting jobs. You get all sorts: glamorous ladies going off to opening nights, posh parties etc; foreign tourists, who are usually very pernickety; actors, musicians and show-biz people of all kinds; also of course, I have a lot of regular clients who come back month after month. People like you to be friendly and chatty and to show an interest in what they want, rather than just force your views on them. You have to be tactful, of course, especially if they want something completely unsuitable. You have to try to head them off discreetly.

There are drawbacks, just as there are in any job. It's very hard work standing all day, and I often have to skip lunch. We open at 9 am and close at 6 pm, so it's a long day. We work Saturdays too, so I suppose it's longer hours than most jobs. On the other hand, the money is good and, of course, I make quite a lot in tips. Not many girls of my age can afford to run a sports car, but I reckon I've worked hard for it.

A salon-owner outlines her career to date.

Ann Stockdale runs Image 8000, a successful beauty and hairdressing salon in Essex, with a partner; she is very experienced in her field, and has a fully rounded knowledge of the beauty, massage and hairdressing business.

Initially, I did a three-year apprenticeship in a hairdressing salon. From junior stylist and improver, I went on to hold a position as a senior stylist, eventually managing a shop in Essex for several years. But fate had a surprise in store for me – in the shape of a broken leg, the result of a skiing holiday. When it healed I had little choice, after such a prolonged absence from the salon I worked in, other than to find another shop to manage. This I did, quite happily, until I married and had my first child. As I went on to have another baby, I was then only able to work on Saturdays. This situation continued for four years, but even working one day a week enabled me to keep up with any new developments in the trade: methods, styles, products etc.

Once the children were at school, it seemed a good idea to work freelance and fit clients in with my daily routine. Life became a little easier when I found myself with a 'set of wheels' and hairdriers etc, although it was hard going, lugging equipment from car to house and back.

I next decided to do beauty therapy, training via the Northern Institute of Massage (postal course). This was an ideal way of learning for me. Each month there were seminars at hotels in London, and the course was completed by a week's intensive training at Blackpool. I started off by using my new-found knowledge at home and then went on to work in a studio for two days a week. Then, after careful consideration and discussion, I decided to go into partnership with a friend. We offer facials, manicures, haircuts, sets and so forth. I also teach meditation once a week, hold a slimming class and do massage, pedicures, and eyebrow plucking. One of the main differences between my salon and many others is that I use only natural products.

This business can be quite demanding; you are, after all, on your feet most of the day. But it is very rewarding. Apart from the more obvious benefits you can offer, such as a new hairstyle or facial 'look', which work wonders for clients' morale, there are the more deep-rooted ones such as the well-being and relaxed feeling that clients can experience from massage.

I thoroughly enjoy my work and can't imagine doing anything else for a living.

Chapter 2
Trichology

Trichology is the study of the hair and scalp. The trichologist specialises in the treatment of diseases and disorders of the hair and scalp and will work either in his or her own clinic, treating patients who come there direct or who are referred by their doctors or hairdressers, or in a clinic attached to a hairdressing salon. All hairdressers are expected to have some knowledge of the subject, so that they can recognise diseases or abnormal conditions and refer them for treatment, but trichology is, in fact, a distinct science and is quite separate from hairdressing.

Training

The recognised qualification in trichology is Membership of the Institute of Trichologists. Minimum requirements are four GCSEs (A–C) or equivalent. English and science subjects are preferred. The course is in two parts, each normally taking one year: the syllabus includes anatomy and physiology, processing of hair, hygiene, massage, nutrition, organic and inorganic chemistry, trichological preparations, micro-diagnostic techniques, electrotherapy, hair and scalp disorders, hair loss, hair care, hirsutism, and the organisation and operation of a trichological practice.

For mature students unable to meet the minimum entry requirements, a Trichological Sciences foundation course is available in some cases which, if satisfied, allows entry to the first-year course. The course is offered at some colleges or can be taken by correspondence.

Students are required to gain some clinical experience before sitting the examinations, and some of this experience must be obtained by attending the Scalp and Hair Hospital in London (228 Stockwell Road, SW9 9SU). Students usually arrange to attend a local clinic on a day or half-day a week basis, and the hospital for a full working week and weekend. Alternative arrangements can be made to suit individual requirements. The range of cases to be seen at the hospital will help the student to appreciate the different techniques that qualified trichologists can use to alleviate the sufferings of those with scalp and hair problems.

It is also possible to study by means of the correspondence course organised by the Institute, which provides tuition specially planned for each grade of study for the Institute's examinations. The course has to be supplemented by practical work, of course, particularly in the latter stages, and advice on this will be given by the Institute.

Many qualified trichologists run their own private practices; others are employed as consultants to industry and the legal profession, or in research and development for cosmetics and pharmaceutical companies.

Some hairdressers take training in trichology as an additional qualification.

Chapter 3
Beauty

Beauty is a much wider and more demanding field than you might imagine. A lot of people have a vague impression that 'beauty' means working in a salon, dabbling about with cosmetics, and that this is a suitable job for those who are too feather-brained or stupid to do anything else.

Nothing could be further from the truth. Beauty work is demanding, calling for a lot of stamina as well as a good level of education. The training for the beauty therapist in particular is far more demanding intellectually than you might imagine and is in some respects akin to nursing. As the comments from our case studies show, you need a real vocation to go into beauty therapy, and you must also be resigned to a lot of ribbing from ignorant friends and even parents who imagine that you are taking up a soft option.

There are various possibilities if you are interested in a career in beauty. If you want a sound training in the full range of beauty treatments, which includes make-up, facial and body massage, electrical epilation (removal of unwanted body hair), slimming treatments etc, then you should take a beauty therapy course. If you are fairly self-confident and interested in selling, you might consider a job as beauty consultant in a department store. There are also other specialisations, eg manicure and make-up, but these on their own offer limited employment opportunities – it is better to take one of these specialist courses as an additional qualification, for example after training as a hairdresser.

Beauty might be thought of as an adjunct to fashion, but in fact a lot of people go into beauty therapy because they are interested in helping people. Beauty treatments and massage are sometimes used to help in the treatment of psychiatric patients, and beauty therapists can also find employment in hospitals working with dermatology or plastic surgery patients, using cosmetic camouflage techniques to help build morale.

19

Beauty Therapist

The beauty therapist, as distinct from the beauty consultant (who usually sells cosmetics in stores), is professionally trained and will usually have a qualification such as the International Beauty Therapist's Diploma.

The work covers a wide spectrum of activities. Facial treatments will include make-up, use of electronic instruments to tighten the muscles of the face, high frequency to stop greasy skin, and cosmetic camouflage following plastic surgery to hide birth-marks or blemishes. There is also a special qualification in electrical epilation: the permanent removal of superfluous hair from face or body. On figure correction treatments, machines now do most of the work and the therapist will be taught how to use them. The title Aesthetician/Aestheticienne is sometimes used for a beauty therapist who is also trained in body massage.

Beauty therapists work in beauty salons or clinics, or on health farms, passenger liners etc. They may also be self-employed, either in their own salons or making home visits to clients. They are not usually employed to sell specific cosmetics or be connected in any way with a particular cosmetic manufacturing company.

The beauty therapist has a good relationship with the medical profession. Many diploma holders work in hospitals performing electrical epilation as dermatologists' assistants, carrying out cosmetic camouflage in association with plastic surgeons or giving facial treatments specifically to help the recovery of mental patients.

Qualities Required

The wide range of treatments demands an extensive knowledge of anatomy, physiology, nutrition and cosmetic science. Sometimes the client will be suffering from a condition that requires medical attention. Therapists have to be able to recognise such a condition and diagnose it accurately, recommending that the client visits a doctor. They also have to decide when a course of treatment should be carried out only with the prior approval of the client's doctor.

Therapists should have a mature, sympathetic personality as well as being attractive and well groomed. They may deal with people who are embarrassed, nervous or suffering from stress, and have to be able to handle them in a kindly and sympathetic way. It is also important to have a confident manner when handling complicated machinery or instruments in order to overcome clients' fears and persuade them to relax.

Training
There are a variety of ways of training as a beauty therapist.

City and Guilds
The City and Guilds of London Institute offers a number of schemes which are currently being revised in the light of changes taking place in the industry. The new developments will provide qualifications on a competence basis to meet the requirements of the Health and Beauty Therapy Training Board (HBTTB) and the National Council for Vocational Qualifications. Most colleges offering City and Guilds schemes require three GCSEs (A–C) including English and a science subject, and some ask for higher qualifications. (See page 64 for details of courses and colleges.)

BTEC (Business & Technology Education Council)
The BTEC National Diploma in Beauty Therapy is a full-time, two-year course available at colleges of further education. Entry qualifications are four GCSEs (A–C) including one subject that demonstrates communication skills, such as English, and another that demonstrates numerical ability, such as maths.

The BTEC Higher National Diploma in Beauty Therapy is also a two-year course which, at the time of writing, is available at only four UK colleges. It is aimed at those who wish to achieve management positions in beauty salons etc, or who wish to run their own businesses. Minimum entry qualifications are one A level, preferably biology, or a BTEC National qualification in a relevant subject. See Part 2 for a list of colleges offering these courses.

There are now also two Higher National Certificates and one National Certificate, which are part-time programmes for people working in this sector.

CIDESCO
CIDESCO (Comité International d'Esthetique et de Cosmetologie) was founded in 1946 to establish international standards of professional ability and integrity. It also aimed at putting members of the various countries in touch with each other for the exchange of professional knowledge and skills. CIDESCO training is available only at a CIDESCO-approved beauty school.

Students must complete a minimum 1,200 hours' attendance at school, which takes 10 months to complete.

Examinations are based on an international syllabus covering all aspects of beauty and are monitored by a CIDESCO delegate. Successful candidates must complete six months' employment working as an aesthetician in a salon before being eligible to receive a diploma. See pp 72–3 for a list of schools which run courses leading to the CIDESCO qualification.

Confederation of International Beauty Therapy and Cosmetology

Courses for the diplomas of the Confederation of International Beauty Therapy and Cosmetology can be taken either in private schools or at a few colleges of further education. To be accepted on a course you need a minimum of three GCSEs, one of which must be English and a second in human biology or another science subject. See Part 2 for details of courses available.

International Health and Beauty Council

The International Health and Beauty Council offers an International Beauty Therapist's Diploma (entry requirements: four GCSEs, A–C) and an International Master's Diploma in Health and Beauty Therapy (entry requirements: two A levels or five GCSEs or equivalent). See Part 2 for a list of courses leading to these diplomas.

International Therapy Examination Council

ITEC is an independent body which offers a variety of certificates and diplomas, including a Beauty Therapy Diploma and an Aestheticienne Diploma. Minimum educational requirement is five GCSEs (A–C), preferably including English language and biology. See pp 86–90 for a list of colleges offering courses.

Beauty Consultant

The main job of the beauty consultant is to sell the products of cosmetics houses. Consultants work mainly in department stores, where they stand behind the counter giving advice on make-up and skin care to customers. They have to be completely familiar with the firm's range of products and must have the confidence and self-assurance to deal with any customer, however difficult.

The consultant usually works on a basic salary, plus commission, and future promotion depends on sales. If you prove to be good at sales you may eventually be promoted to senior consultant, with the job of visiting the various stores to supervise the other consultants, training newcomers and making sure that their counter displays and personal appearance are up to standard. You will be expected to help in-store promotions and, if you are interested and ambitious, might eventually aim for a job in marketing.

When an important new product is launched, the consultants are called into the head office to hear all about it and be instructed in its proper use. They may also be asked for their comments on current lines and customer reaction.

A good consultant may also be promoted to demonstrator, with the job of travelling round the country giving public demonstrations on make-up and skin care in stores, schools, women's clubs, colleges etc.

Qualities Required

The beauty consultant need not be a raving beauty, but she should be extremely well groomed and have a pleasant and attractive manner. In fact, she has to be an advertisement for the products she is trying to sell, and being a good saleswoman is an important part of the job. It is also important to have a genuine interest in other people and to be able to listen attentively and sympathetically to their problems.

Training

All the main cosmetic manufacturers run special courses for beauty consultants, but they are not usually open to school-leavers. These short, intensive courses are usually designed for girls in their early twenties who already have some selling experience, preferably on the cosmetics counter of a large chemist's shop or department store. The minimum age to be accepted is 18, and more mature entrants are preferred. If you are younger, it may be easier to find a job in the general cosmetics or perfumery department of a large store or chemist's shop or take a Saturday job while still studying. There you will become familiar with the range of goods available and learn how to deal with customers' queries. After some general experience in selling you can then apply to the cosmetics houses. The best policy is simply to write to the firms of your choice, who will then arrange to interview you. Once accepted, you are given several weeks of intensive training before being appointed to a store. At first you might be working with an experienced consultant who knows the ropes, but after a few months you will probably be on your own. If you wish to take a college course (it is not strictly necessary but may be helpful), the following are available:

1. The International Health and Beauty Council awards a Beauty Consultant's Certificate, for which two GCSEs (A–C) are required. Candidates must be at least 18 or must be taking the course in conjunction with another approved course or must be employed in a store, by a cosmetics house or in a hairdressing or beauty salon. See Part 2 for a list of colleges running courses for this certificate.
2. The International Therapy Examination Council offers a Beauty Consultancy Certificate, and again you must be 18 by the time you sit the exam. Entrance qualifications vary with the individual college, but two GCSEs (A–C) are usually asked for. See Part 2 for a list of colleges offering courses.

Beautician

The beautician specialises in skin care. Her work includes cleansing the skin, make-up, removing blemishes and helping the client to counteract the effects of tension and fatigue. This includes massage of the face, either by hand or electricity, removal of superfluous hair and broken veins, manicures and pedicures, shaping eyebrows and colouring eyelashes, acne and open pore treatment, make-up for special occasions and make-up lessons. In a large establishment there will be beauticians who specialise in electrolysis and manicure.

The work of the beautician and of the beauty therapist often overlap, but the beautician is not concerned with body treatments and her training does not include such an exacting knowledge of anatomy and physiology.

The beautician works in a salon which may be part of a larger establishment: beauty salons are now to be found in hairdressing establishments, department stores or in the growing number of health farms, health clubs etc. On the whole, however, job opportunities are not particularly good for beauticians, as most salons and health farms prefer the wider expertise offered by the beauty therapist.

Qualities Required

The beautician must have a calm and even temperament, a cheerful outgoing personality and an attractive, well-groomed appearance. It is not necessary to be young and beautiful – in fact, many employers prefer their staff to be older and more mature – but you do need to have a good appearance. Good grooming and good health are essential; it also helps to have supple, well-kept hands. After all, no client will have much confidence in the advice of a beautician who is herself spotty and badly groomed, with bitten fingernails. Relaxation is usually an essential part of the treatment, so the beautician must also have a positive, reassuring manner that inspires confidence.

Training

The Confederation of International Beauty Therapy and Cosmetology, the International Health and Beauty Council and the International Therapy Examination Council offer courses for beauticians. See Part 2 for a list of schools running these courses.

Manicurist

Manicure is the specialised care and treatment of the hands. Manicurists massage the hands, treat the skin around the nails, look after the condition of the cuticles, and shape the nails. They usually also varnish the nails. Manicurists are employed in hairdressing salons, beauty salons and health clinics.

Training

Manicure is usually included as part of the training for a beautician or beauty therapist, but for those who want to specialise it is possible to take it as a separate qualification. The International Health and Beauty Council and the International Therapy Examination Council both offer separate Manicure Certificates (see pp 77 and 86). Colleges of further education often offer the City and Guilds course, usually in conjunction with a hairdressing or beauty course.

Electrolysist

The electrolysist specialises in epilation, which is the removal of superfluous hair from face and body by means of electricity. The trained operator works either in a specialist clinic (such as the Tao Clinic) or in a beauty clinic.

Training

Electrolysis is part of the training of the beauty therapist but it can also be taken as a specialist qualification. The Confederation of International Beauty Therapy and Cosmetology, the International Health and Beauty Council and the International Therapy Examination Council all offer certificates or diplomas in Electrolysis. You need three to five GCSEs (A–C) for entry to the courses. See Part 2 for a list of colleges offering courses.

The Institute of Electrolysis offers a diploma. No specific educational qualifications are required, just a good general standard of education (see p 92).

Private Schools and Colleges of Further Education

Colleges of further education offer beauty courses leading to recognised qualifications, and you can be reasonably certain that the standard of tuition, facilities etc will be satisfactory. More and more colleges are now offering courses in beauty therapy, and it is advisable to check, before contacting private schools, whether the course you are interested in is available at a local college.

Private schools are expensive. A course that includes a CIDESCO qualification will cost at least £4,500 plus VAT. Short courses are considerably cheaper but the training provided may not be widely accepted in the industry.

Choose a recognised course, leading to one of the following qualifications:

City and Guilds
BTEC
SCOTVEC
CIDESCO
CIBTC
IHBC
ITEC

NCVQ accredited examinations will eventually supersede most of the above but entrants to the industry requiring an internationally recognised qualification may continue to need a more exam-focused assessment..

Some beauty schools offer their own diplomas, which may be of dubious standard and of little use for getting employment in the industry.

Schools which demand higher entry qualifications (GCSEs, A levels or equivalent) are likely to be of a higher standard. Try to find a course which offers as comprehensive a range of subjects as possible.

The Park School of Beauty Therapy, Storcroft House, London Road, Retford, Nottinghamshire DN22 7EB runs full-time and part-time courses, ranging from a few weeks' to two years' duration. The School's courses vary in emphasis, some stressing the academic and others a more practical approach.

Case Studies

What do students think of private schools? We interviewed three students at the Beauty Clinic in London and asked them for their views on the course.

Fiona (aged 19)

I decided fairly early on that I wanted three things from any course I did: it should equip me with a skill, it should be creative, and it should have some medical content.

My first choice was speech therapy, but I had the wrong A levels. It's very difficult to make the right choice, and you don't really get much help. When I was 16 or so I wanted to be a nurse, for example, but I realise now I would have made a very bad nurse. It shouldn't be necessary to make a career choice so early – lots of people just don't know their minds at that age.

I was very lucky because I took a year off after school, and it did help me to think about things and decide what I would really like to do. I would advise everyone to do that, if they possibly can. It helps you to grow up a bit and find out what life is like outside the school gate. Some of the girls on the course have gone under because they came here straight from school and they simply were not dedicated enough. They had this glamorous image in their minds, and of course it was a let-down when they got here and found it was all hard work.

It was a surprise to find out how academic the course was, particularly the science content. Intellectually it has been much harder than I expected. But no-one should let that put them off, because they start you off right from scratch. You do have to put in quite a lot of work in the evening, which cuts down on your social life a bit, and if you do have too many late nights it's difficult to concentrate when you are trying to study.

My advice to anyone thinking of this career would be to think hard about it first, to make sure you have the necessary dedication. Then, having made up your mind, don't let yourself be put off by the mockery – there tends to be a general feeling that this is a non-job and you have to do a lot of explaining that it is *not* simply a case of slapping on make-up all day.

Claire (aged 22)

I had no idea what I wanted to do, except that I wanted to work with people. The careers advice at our school was really bad. There was a tremendous amount of pressure put on you to *decide* something, even when you felt you weren't ready for it. The careers teacher didn't want to know about people who had no idea at all what they wanted to do. As you grow older and your school career is coming to an end, there is this horrible feeling that the options are all closing and authority is washing its hands of you if you can't make up your mind.

I know I wasn't capable of deciding anything like that at 16. Even if I had decided something it would probably have been wrong, as I have changed so much in the interval. You really do grow up a lot in that first couple of years after leaving school. A year off after school to make up your mind about the future would be a very good idea for most people, I think.

I did two years in catering after school. It seems a big jump, I know, from catering to beauty therapy, but the similarity in the two jobs is the contact with people. That was what attracted me to catering, but it was the responsibility I couldn't handle. I was always vaguely aware of beauty therapy as a possibility, but it took me ages to find out about it. There really is a great dearth of information about this field and most people tend to imagine it consists of doing make-up all day. I had to do a lot of scratching around for information, finding out about the various courses and asking around to find out what was the best school.

Oh yes, I am absolutely convinced now that I have done the right thing. I am enjoying the course very much, and I think the school gives you tremendous training. It was a surprise to me how serious it all was and how thoroughly they went into things. I would like to have my own business eventually – probably that will mean working from home at first, but I won't mind that. I would like to travel too – to Australia or Canada if I could get a work permit. The thought of working on the Continent doesn't attract me at all because of the language problem.

Jane (aged 18)

Like Fiona, I found I had the wrong A levels when it came to choosing a career. I had wanted to do occupational therapy, but I had to think again. I chose this because there is a family connection: my mother worked in beauty and in hairdressing, so I did have a fairly good idea of what I was going into. She's green with envy, actually, at the thought of the training I'm getting here. The school was quite helpful, once I had decided on this as a career. It supplied me with a list of beauty schools and I just wrote around. I think I was very lucky to get taken on here. You're given a good training and lots of individual attention, which you wouldn't get in a college. It's good fun too, which I hadn't expected.

The course certainly educates you in a general sense. I'm far more aware of the importance of diet and exercise, for example, and you learn a lot about bringing up children, and nutrition, and the diseases people are prone to. In a way, it's rather like a finishing school with a vocation at the end of it.

I'd love to do TV make-up afterwards, but you need to have a hairdressing qualification as well, and I don't fancy that. I think I might eventually specialise in cosmetic surgery – hospital work would be fascinating and the whole thing has a tremendous appeal.

I agree that you have to be dedicated. The course does involve a lot of hard work, and it can be difficult to buckle down to it after the long hard slog through school. It can come as a surprise too, because people have this feather-brained image of the job. I had to put up with a lot of teasing at school when I announced what I was going to do. The girls used to say things like, 'Why don't you start on yourself first?' and stuff like that. You have to be determined not to be mocked and just get it across to people that this is a serious job.

TV Work

A lot of people who go in for beauty training are keen to work in television, attracted by what seems to be a glamorous and exciting life. But they should be aware that there are drawbacks: the competition is obviously very fierce, and the hours are irregular – you will often be required to work over weekends and bank holidays. Also TV companies are taking on fewer and fewer make-up artists because films are increasingly being produced by independent film-makers operating on a contract basis. At the same time there is a plentiful supply of people in television with basic skills including wigmaking which covers maintenance, repair and dressing, thus making a qualification in beauty culture and hairdressing almost redundant.

The London College of Fashion offers courses that combine beauty culture and hairdressing. A three-year Hairdressing and Beauty Therapy Diploma provides a foundation in all aspects of hairdressing with the addition of Afro hair techniques. To qualify you must be at least 16 years of age and have obtained at least one of the following: a BTEC First Certificate or Diploma; a minimum of four GCSEs (or equivalent), including English language, a biological science and preferably maths; a full CPVE Certificate with an appropriate profile; a BTEC 14–16 preparatory programme Certificate of Achievement and an appropriate profile. The syllabus covers hairdressing, wigmaking and all aspects of beauty therapy.

A two-year full-time course leading to a BTEC Higher National Diploma in Design Fashion Styling for Hair and Make-up is also available from the London College of Fashion. You must be 18 and have achieved at least one of the following: four GCSE passes and art at A level; a BTEC Diploma in a relevant area; a foundation course.

For further information write to The School of Fashion Promotion, 20 John Prince's Street, London W1M 0BJ, or ring 071-629 9401.

Chapter 4
Massage

Introduction

Massage can be described as the manipulation of the soft tissues of the body. It is one of the oldest known forms of healing – not only was it used by the Greeks and Romans, it is known that massage therapy was used by the Chinese centuries before that. For thousands of years massage has been used to alleviate pain, tone up muscles, improve general fitness and bring back elasticity to joints.

Basically there are two types of massage: remedial massage which is used for its therapeutic value on muscles and joints after illness or injury, and body massage which is used for its general toning effect after Turkish baths, sauna baths etc. Whatever kind of massage is used, its application is a skilled art which should be performed only by a competent therapist.

Qualities Required

There is much more to massage than the ability to use your hands well. You must understand basic anatomy and physiology, so that you will understand the benefits of massage on the human body, eg as an aid to digestion, circulation, nervous tension etc. You must also know just when – and why – massage is *not* advisable in certain cases. You must understand the value of sauna, Turkish and steam baths and other types of remedial baths, and be able to operate the equipment, such as infra-red and ultra-violet lamps, faradic muscle-toning equipment, vibrators and vacusage machines.

You must possess a good understanding of the muscular system so that you thoroughly appreciate, and can advise on and provide, the right procedure for specific results. You will be required to offer guidance to clients who wish to add or lose inches, gain in muscle tone and definition, or achieve a feeling of all-round fitness.

You should understand, too, about dietetics, so that you can appreciate the value of certain foods and how diet can affect health and fitness.

Above all, you must have a calm, confident manner that will create confidence in your clients. Many will be in pain, or suffering from stress and anxiety. You will have to be able to allay their fears and set their minds at rest.

Opportunities

With the trend towards a sensible pursuit of body fitness and appearance, there is an ever-increasing need for trained people who can create confidence in clients and who can provide a skilled professional service in the massage establishment.

Massage staff are employed in health hydros, nature cure clinics, health farms etc, where they often work in collaboration with osteopaths and other therapists. Turkish baths and saunas, which can now be found all over the country, also employ masseurs, and many local authorities have installed saunas in their public baths or sports centres, usually with massage provided. In addition, massage is usually an important aspect of the treatment in beauty salons and slimming clinics.

As well as these various openings, many people set up their own private practices after training, often working in close collaboration with local doctors who may send them patients. Training usually includes the recognition of certain symptoms and diseases which should be referred in the first instance to the patient's doctor. Massage treatment in these cases should be carried out only with the approval of the doctor.

Training

Body massage is usually regarded as part of the training for an aestheticienne or beauty therapist, and is included in the syllabus for the diplomas of the Confederation of International Beauty Therapy and Cosmetology, the International Health and Beauty Council and the International Therapy Examination Centre (see Part 2).

The International Institute of Sports Therapy, a branch of the International Health and Beauty Council, is currently being sponsored by the EC to set up examinations in massage across Europe.

The Northern Institute of Massage provides specialised

training. It offers two course programmes: one in body massage and physical culture for the student who wants a career in sauna or Turkish bath etc, where there is a demand for massage services; one in remedial massage for students who want to work in health hydros and similar establishments, as assistants to practising therapists, with sports clubs or in private practice.

There are no entry requirements for the Northern Institute's training courses, apart from being 18 or over at the date of enrolment. Students are taken on a one-month trial basis.

The Northern Institute specialises in a format of training combining approved home-study correspondence tuition linked to short-period practical class instruction at the relevant stages of training. The college has been accredited by the Council for the Accreditation of Correspondence Colleges. Successful graduates receive the Institute's diploma. See Part 2 for further details of the courses.

Aromatherapy

Aromatherapy is increasing in popularity, in this country as well as abroad. Some aromatherapists have their own consulting rooms. Health spas, clubs and some of the larger beauty salons also offer the treatment.

Aromatherapy relaxes muscles, reduces tension; it is used by practitioners of complementary medicine, and as an adjunct to orthodox medicine provided that the presiding GP has overall control. Specialists claim that cellulite deposits can be broken down, and sinus problems and acne can be counteracted. Those who experience the treatment speak glowingly of the relaxed, luxurious and sensual feeling aromatherapy generates.

Technique

Treatment involves two techniques: first, massage with essential oils selected from fruits, flowers, plants and grasses. Over 100 different oils are available and many aromatherapists make up their own blend. Each has a different function: for instance, rose is antidepressant, citrus oils stimulate the circulation, and lavender is cleansing and antiseptic. Inhalation of the aromas is the second part of the technique.

If the symptom is general tiredness or a run-down feeling, a good aromatherapist will select the appropriate oils to combat the problem. Oil is distributed all over the body by basic massage strokes, and acupuncture points receive certain techniques.

Training

Aromatherapy can be studied at many colleges throughout the country. The International Federation of Aromatherapists, Royal Masonic Hospital, Ravenscourt Park, London W6 0TN, is the only independent professional body representing aromatherapists in the UK. The IFA sets standards for teaching aromatherapy as well as for individual aromatherapists, and acts as an information service for the press and the general public. Aromatherapy courses following the guidelines set out in the IFA's syllabus for training are accredited by the IFA from whom a list of accredited colleges can be obtained if you send £1 (either in stamps or by cheque) plus an sae.

A 10-day diploma course, which provides training in massage based on the original Marguerite Maury method, is offered by Aromatherapy Associates Ltd, 68 Maltings Place, London SW6 2BY; 071-731 8129. Students must be at least 20 years old and be qualified therapists with a recognised diploma in anatomy and physiology.

The International Therapy Examination Council provides a list of tutors and schools teaching aromatherapy to international standards.

Reflexology

Reflexology is a pressure therapy of the feet used 2,500 years ago by the Egyptians and today for promoting well-being and relieving pain. It is practised by many aromatherapists; it is based on the principle that the feet contain hundreds of minute pressure points and when a firm controlled pressure is applied it has a stimulating effect on the entire system.

If there is a dysfunction in the body, the feet reflect this by showing a sensitivity in the corresponding reflex point. The entire structure and functioning of the body is reflected within the feet; when pressure is applied a stimulation through the nerve pathways is created, thereby relieving pain, improving nerve and blood supply and normalising the entire body.

Technique

Sessions last around 40 minutes. The reflexologist makes a detailed examination of the soles of the feet with her thumbs and fingers. Particularly tender reflexes can be related to bodily problems. Appropriate areas are then treated; this is very relaxing.

As a diagnostic 'probe', reflexology can be surprisingly accurate. Although it should not be taken as a substitute for medical treatment, it certainly reduces physical tension. Those who have participated claim it is an excellent anti-stress treatment, and experience a feeling of well-being.

For further information on reflexology contact the British School of Reflexology, Holistic Healing Centre, 92 Old Sheering Road, Old Harlow, Essex CM17 0JW.

Reflexology is also offered as an examination subject by the International Therapy Examination Council (see Part 2).

Case Studies
Felicity Young, remedial masseuse

The most important thing about this job is that you *must* have a sense of vocation. It comes under the heading of medicine, because most of the people you see have something wrong with them and you must have an interest in helping them. It's like nursing too, in that a good masseuse is born, not made. Either you can do it or you can't, for massage is very much an art or skill. You need to have a certain sensitivity – you have to be able to *feel* what is wrong.

I did my training at the Northern Institute of Massage and it was interesting that most of us doing the training had some trouble of our own and that was what had impelled us into doing it. Originally I trained as a librarian, but then I developed back trouble and needed treatment. That was what first aroused my interest in remedial massage; once I realised how people could be helped I decided to do the Northern Institute training.

Once I had been accepted as a student I gave up my job and took a part-time job as a telephonist so that I would be free to do the studying required.

After I trained I found this job in Mary's clinic. She concentrates on using her Ionar machine (see below) and I do most of the massage. That's the hardest part of this job – to get started – and it's probably easiest to join someone else's clinic and build up a clientèle that way. You could probably find a job quite easily in a beauty salon or a sauna establishment, but it's not the same. You have to remember that remedial massage is very different from the kind of massage you would get in a beauty clinic. It calls for real strength and hard work.

Almost all my clients have something wrong with them – back problems, tennis elbow, arthritis etc – very few have massage just because they think it would be a nice thing to do. Most people are walking around with something wrong with them. They only notice it when inflammation develops and it starts to hurt. Mary, my partner, tells this lovely story about a patient who had one leg an inch shorter than the other. It had been like that for 18 years and she asked him how on earth he managed. It was quite simple, he said; he had just had all his trousers altered to fit when he bought them. Well, Mary told him, you are going to have a problem when you go home tonight. I've straightened you out now and both legs are the same length again!

I treat on average six patients a day - it's fairly tiring and that is really quite a heavy work-load. The treatment for each patient takes about an hour.

I believe in being very informal with the clients - I find it helps them to relax. If you have too clinical an atmosphere it can be very off-putting. We usually give the clients a cup of tea at the end of the session and they can sit and chat to the other patients coming in and out. People coming for the first time are usually very nervous and apprehensive about what is going to happen to them: an informal atmosphere reassures them.

Mary James, remedial masseuse and therapist

I would think this is a very good time for young people to go into massage as a career. There is far more interest in it now and the public tends to have far more understanding of its remedial value. Massage used to be a word that made people snigger and I suppose the more ignorant ones still do; it still has a slight connotation. But massage is a serious job, and the more people take it up as a career, the more seriously it will be treated. What is marvellous is that you can go on to more and more advanced work, treating people with injuries and eventually going on to osteopathy.

I concentrate now on giving treatments with the Ionar machine, which aids healing with pulsed electro-magnetic energy. It works by putting back energy into the cells of the body when the cells have suffered shock or damage. The great thing is that it does this without inducing heat in the tissues, so you can't burn. In fact, it is 100 per cent safe. What it really does is to make the body heal itself if an organ is sick or infected. It can speed up healing by up to 40 per cent, especially bone damage; it can even work through a plaster cast.

Chapter 5

Health Studios and Slimming Clinics

The last few years have seen a great upsurge of interest in health and fitness. Everyone now wants to be fit and slim, and this has resulted in a boom in the number of health clubs, slimming clinics, exercise classes and beauty farms. Most of these are unisex, and cater for people of all ages.

Health Studios

One recent development is the 'health studio', usually unisex, which offers a whole range of activities. Most popular are the classes in body-conditioning – usually to jazz or rock music. There is a tremendous number of these classes now available; some are very similar to 'keep-fit' classes while others are more akin to modern dance routines. You can find classes in the Californian work-out, New York stretch, keep-fit jazz, body-conditioning, body stretch, slow stretch, body toning, disco keep-fit, funky exercises, modern ballet, tap-dancing, yoga, classical Indian dance, self-defence and aerobics. The real enthusiasts go to classes every day, often in their lunch hour, while others might go once or twice a week. The exercises are designed to shape, tone and stretch the body, enabling the client to feel fitter, look slimmer and be healthier. Almost all exercises are done to music and clients may progress from beginner's grade up to the more advanced (and difficult) exercises.

Most studios also offer advice on diet and home exercises.

Job Opportunities
Generally, beauty clubs, exercise clubs and health studios are established and run by people who have training either in beauty therapy, massage, ballet, yoga or modern dancing. Some have qualifications in several different disciplines, or may have taken up health and beauty after a successful career as a dancer or

model. Depending on the facilities offered by the particular clinic or studio, staff employed will be required to have qualifications in beauty therapy, yoga, dancing, hairdressing, manicure etc. (See Part 2 for qualifications available.)

Obviously, to work in this field you have to be extremely fit and healthy, with a keen interest in keeping yourself in shape. It helps too to have an interest in other people and a real desire to help them. People going to a class for the first time are usually very shy and self-conscious (especially if they are seriously overweight or out of condition), and it will be your job to put them at ease and help them to relax and enjoy the exercises. If it is too painful, exhausting and humiliating the client is unlikely to come back for more. You will also have to recognise when a client has a serious health problem and should be referred to a doctor.

Training

Some of the big studios take on students who want to become qualified in a particular 'method'. It is not necessary to have done any previous training, though you must obviously be young and fit. Training can take from six months to a year, depending on how much time you can devote to classes. Courses can be shorter if you are prepared to do intensive training.

Students who have successfully qualified will probably be taken on as full-time or part-time teachers, or else helped to find posts elsewhere.

You can, of course, go on to qualify in other 'methods' or take supplementary training in ballet, yoga, massage etc, to increase your expertise. In this field, the more versatile you are the better, so far as employment prospects are concerned. (Many studios offer a wide range of classes in dance, yoga and the various 'methods' of body conditioning.)

For training and qualifications available in beauty therapy, massage etc, see Part 2 of this book.

Slimming Clinics

Health clubs and exercise studios aim to control weight through exercise and diet. Slimming clinics tend to concentrate on passive exercise through the use of machines. Machines such as the Slendertone machines and gyratory massagers are used to tone and tighten muscles, break down fatty tissue and disperse excess fluid. Some beauty clinics and health clubs also offer this as part of the service. In addition, they usually also offer advice on nutrition, sensible eating and home exercise.

Job Opportunities
The range of jobs available will depend very much on the facilities offered by the particular clinic. A clinic that concentrates purely on spot-reducing will want staff to operate the various machines. A firm such as Slendertone Ltd offers a two-day training in the use of its ultra-tone range, free of charge if you buy one of the machines. Other clinics will also employ staff with qualifications in beauty therapy, massage, manicure and pedicure. See Part 2 for the various qualifications and training available.

Professional Organisations

The International Council of Health, Fitness and Sports Therapists (ICHFST), 38a Portsmouth Road, Woolston, Southampton SO2 5AD is the umbrella organisation for all the qualified professionals in the health, fitness and sports therapy industries. It covers the Finnish Sauna Society (FSS) and the Institute for Massage and Movement (IMM). Membership of all of the above is at three grades – associates, members and fellows – and services provided include advice on legal and employment issues, preferential insurance terms, publications and seminars.

Chapter 6

Applying for a Job

To be successful in applying for jobs it is most important to be organised right from the start. Look on it as a plan of campaign in which each step – letter of application, curriculum vitae, employer's application form, interview – must be carried out carefully and enthusiastically.

Take time to write a good letter of application, and ask a friend to vet it for spelling mistakes. Make your curriculum vitae (see below) as neat and tidy as you can, and make sure you have included all the facts.

For jobs in this field the interview is crucial. You may have very impressive academic qualifications and you may have acquired all sorts of certificates and diplomas, but your manner, your personal appearance and how you conduct yourself at the interview will be vital. However, don't allow yourself to get into a panic about interviews. See the checklist of points to remember for interviews on p 43.

Remember too that there is a technique to conducting interviews. This is explained further on in this chapter. Once you know what the pattern is and what to expect, you will find interviews far less frightening.

Letter of Application

□ Do a rough draft of the letter first to make sure that you have covered all essential points.
□ Give details of your qualifications and experience (your curriculum vitae) on a separate sheet.
□ Make absolutely sure that there are no spelling mistakes or grammatical errors in your letter. If in any doubt, ask a friend to look it over for you.
□ Use good quality writing-paper for your letter.

☐ Keep your letter brief and to the point. Mention where you saw the advertisement.
☐ Keep a copy of your letter for reference.

Curriculum Vitae

See the following page for how to lay out your curriculum vitae. It should give:

☐ full name and address
☐ date of birth
☐ schools attended
☐ examinations passed
☐ any other honours won at school
☐ any particular position of authority held at scnool, eg school captain
☐ training courses or colleges attended and qualifications gained
☐ previous jobs held or any other experience gained
☐ present employment, it any
☐ names and addresses of two referees. One of these should be a previous employer or someone who has personal knowledge of your capabilities.
☐ personal interests/hobbies
☐ languages. If you have adequate written or speaking knowledge of any languages, mention it here.
☐ if you have a current driving licence mention it here.

The Interview

You will find interviews less frightening if you remember that all interviews have a pattern.

1. The interviewer may start by putting you at your ease, making small talk about the weather or your journey to the interview.
2. He or she will then try to draw you out by asking about your career to date, what you have been doing since you left school etc. The interviewer wants you to talk so as to get an impression of your manner with people, but beware of rambling on for too long.
3. The interviewer will then probably move on to your letter or application form and go over the details. It is important not to become bored or irritated at this point. All the things being asked may already be there on the form, but give the details again, politely.
4. Have an answer ready when you are asked how you see your career developing, or what you would like to be doing in five years' time.
5. Be ready for the question, 'Why are you applying for this particular

MARY BROWN
32 PARK AVENUE, MANCHESTER M3 5AW

Tel: 061-123 4567

DATE OF BIRTH: ....

AGE NOW: ....

SCHOOLS ATTENDED:

(Name and town)   (From) — (To)

COLLEGES ATTENDED:

(Name and town)   (From) — (To)

QUALIFICATIONS:

(Name of examination)   (Subject)   (Grade)

(Include all school/college examinations which you have passed and any other qualifications/certificates you have which you think would be relevant or of interest to employers)

POSITIONS HELD:

INTERESTS AND ACTIVITIES:

FURTHER EDUCATIONAL PLANS:

EXPERIENCE:

REFERENCES:

(1) (Name of referee)   (Address)   (Tel no)

(2)

(3)

A sample curriculum vitae

job?' Even if you have been sent by an agency you must still make it sound as if *you* are keen on the job and want to apply for it.

6. The interviewer will probably then ask if you have a clear picture of the job and what it entails. This is to see if you have really thought about it.

7. At the end, the interviewer will probably ask if *you* have any questions, and you must try to think of something to say. If it looks as if you are going to be offered the job, this could be the point to clear up anything you are not sure about. We give below some points to watch under 'Accepting a Job'. This would be the moment to ask to see where you are going to work, if you have not already done so, and to clear up any queries about salary, holidays, pension rights etc.

Checklist of Points to Remember

Remember that for most jobs your appearance, manner and general level of education will be as important as your diplomas.

☐ Be on time for the interview. If you are even five minutes late it will be a black mark against you, so leave in plenty of time, allowing for traffic jams, trains being late etc.

☐ *It is essential to be well groomed* – immaculate make-up, tidy hair, clean hands and nails, clean shoes.

☐ Dress neatly rather than flashily. Avoid heavy fragrances or low necklines. Whatever you wear should be clean and well pressed.

☐ Smile pleasantly and look directly at the interviewer.

☐ Don't smoke even if invited to do so.

☐ Speak clearly without mumbling. Don't say 'sort of' or 'you know' every other word. Your voice will be important.

☐ Don't giggle or make jokey remarks.

☐ Be honest about your abilities.

☐ Don't allow yourself to get angry or irritated at anything the interviewer says. He or she may be finding out how well you stand up to pressure. Try to keep cool and unfussed no matter how the conversation goes.

☐ Try to avoid giving 'yes' and 'no' answers, but on the other hand don't ramble.

☐ Remember that you have to sell yourself to the employer. Talk about your good points and what you can do, rather than what you can't do.

☐ Above all, try to appear interested in the job. The employer will always prefer someone who seems lively and enthusiastic.

Telephone Interviews

There is an increasing trend towards telephone interviewing. If the employer likes the sound of you during the preliminary interview by telephone, you will be asked to come along for a more formal interview. It is most important that you should be well prepared for this.

- ☐ Write out all the relevant details about yourself on a piece of paper in case you become flustered – school, exams passed, qualifications for the job, training courses completed etc.
- ☐ Try to speak in a firm, clear voice. Don't mumble and 'um' and 'er' and say 'sort of' and 'you know' every other word. Your voice is the only thing the employer has to go on, so you must try to sound pleasant, self-assured and capable. Take a deep breath and try not to gabble through being nervous.
- ☐ Come straight to the point. 'I'm ringing about the advertisement in today's paper. It sounds very interesting. Could you tell me more about it please?'
- ☐ If you are ringing from a pay phone, make sure you have an ample supply of coins, or buy a Phonecard and go to a Phonecard telephone.

Checklist of Questions to be Prepared for

The interviewer is sure to ask some, if not all, of these questions – make sure you have answers prepared.

- ☐ What made you decide to go in for this career?
- ☐ What made you apply for this job?
- ☐ What makes you think you will be good at it?
- ☐ What particularly attracts you about this job?
- ☐ How would you like your career to develop?/What would you like to be doing in five years' time?
- ☐ What do you like doing in your spare time?
- ☐ Tell me about your family.
- ☐ (if you already have a job) Why do you want to leave your present job?

Accepting a Job

Before you write a letter of acceptance, you should make sure you know your position. No one should accept a job without understanding what the job entails, what the hours and rate of pay are and what the holiday entitlement is. If you have any doubts or queries, now is the time to clear them up. It is no use saying later that you didn't realise what the job involved, or that you thought you were entitled to four weeks' holiday when it turns out to be two.

Contract of Employment

A contract of employment exists as soon as someone offers you a job (even verbally) at a certain rate of pay and you accept. Within 13 weeks of your starting work the employer is required by law to give you written details of your contract. These include:

☐ job title
☐ pay
☐ how you are paid (weekly, monthly etc)
☐ hours of work
☐ holiday entitlement and pay
☐ length of notice
☐ disciplinary and grievance procedures
☐ pension schemes
☐ any requirement to join a specific trade union.

If you are not given a copy of your contract within 13 weeks of joining a firm, you should ask for it. The contract of employment could be important to you later, so make sure that you keep it in a safe place.

Part 2

Chapter 7

Courses and Qualifications Available

Hairdressing

City and Guilds of London Institute
46 Britannia Street, London WC1X 9RG; 071-278 2468

The NVQ system of awards, currently being developed by the City and Guilds of London Institute and the Hairdressing Training Board, covers areas of work at specific levels of achievement. Each area contains a series of units which may be tackled in any order, depending on the needs of the individual. Trainees are thus able to progress at their own speed and are assessed when they are ready. Success in a range of units, which is assessed in the workplace, supported by written and oral work, leads to a Record of Achievements.

As the NVQs become accredited, some of the following qualifications currently being offered by the City and Guilds Institute may be phased out. At present they are:

(a) Introduction to Salon Services (3570)
(b) Advanced Studies In Hairdressing (3000)
(c) Salon Management (3060)

The following colleges offer one or more of the above courses. Please contact them direct for up-to-date information.

Local Authority Colleges

Avon
City of Bath College
Avon Street
Bath BA1 1UP
0225 312191

Brunel College
Ashley Down, Bristol BS7 9BU
0272 241241

West of England College
The Manor
Brewery Lane
Holcombe
Bath BA3 53G
0761 232757

Weston-super-Mare College
Knightstone Road
Weston-super-Mare BS23 2AL
0934 621301

Bedfordshire
Barnfield College
New Bedford Road, Luton
LU3 2AX
0582 507531

Bedford College
Cauldwell Street, Bedford
MK42 5AH
0234 345151

Berkshire
Langley College
Station Road, Langley
Slough SL3 8BY
0753 49222

Reading College
Crescent Road, Reading RG1 5RQ
0734 583501

Buckinghamshire
Aylesbury College
Oxford Road, Aylesbury
HP21 8PD
0296 434111

Milton Keynes College
Woughton Centre
Chaffron Way
Leadenhall West
Milton Keynes MK6 5LP
0908 668998

Cambridgeshire
Cambridge College
Newmarket Road
Cambridge CB1 2NA
0223 357545

Isle College
Ramnoth Road, Wisbech
PE13 2JE
0945 582561/5

Peterborough College
Park Crescent, Peterborough
PE1 4DZ
0733 67366

Channel Isles
Guernsey College
Route Des Coutanchez
St Peter Port, Guernsey
0481 727121

Highlands College
St Saviour
Jersey
0534 71800

Cheshire
Halton College
Kingsway, Widnes
WA8 7QQ
051-423 1391

North Cheshire College
Warrington North Campus
Winwick Road, Warrington
WA2 8QA
0925 814343

South Cheshire College
Dane Bank Avenue, Crewe
CW2 8AB
0270 69133

South Trafford College
Manchester Road, West
Timperley
Altrincham WA14 5PQ
061-973 7064

West Cheshire College
Regent Street
Ellesmere Port
South Wirral L65 8EJ
051-356 2300

Cleveland
Hartlepool College
Stockton Street
Hartlepool TS24 7NT
0429 275453

Kirby College
Roman Road
Middlesbrough TS5 5PJ
0642 813706

Cornwall
Cornwall College
Redruth TR15 3RD
0209 712911

St Austell College
Palace Road, St Austell
PL25 4BW
0726 67911

Saltash College
Church Road
Saltash PL12 4AE
0752 844777

Cumbria
Barrow-in-Furness College
Howard Street
Barrow-in-Furness LA14 1NB
0229 825017

Carlisle College
Victoria Place
Carlisle CA1 1HS
0228 24464

Kendal College
Milnthorpe Road, Kendal
LA9 5AY
0539 724313

West Cumbria College
Park Lane, Workington
CA14 2RW
0900 64331

Derbyshire
Chesterfield College
Infirmary Road
Chesterfield S41 7NG
0246 231212

Derby College
Prince Charles Avenue
Mackworth
Derby DE3 4LR
0332 519951

High Peak College
Harpur Hill
Buxton SK17 9JZ
0298 71100

North Derbyshire Tertiary
College
Rectory Road
Clowne, Nr Chesterfield S43 4BQ
0246 810332

Devon
East Devon College
Bolham Road
Tiverton EX16 6SH
0884 254247

Exeter College
Hele Road
Exeter EX4 4JS
0392 273071

North Devon College
Old Sticklepath Hill
Barnstaple EX31 2BQ
0271 45291

Plymouth College
Kings Road
Devonport, Plymouth PL1 5QG
0752 385314

South Devon College
Newton Road
Torquay TQ2 5BY
0803 213242

Dorset
Bournemouth and Poole College
Landsdowne
Bournemouth BH1 3JJ
0202 295511

Weymouth College
Cranford Avenue
Weymouth DT4 7LQ
0305 761100

Durham
Bishop Auckland College
Woodhouse Lane
Bishop Auckland DL14 6JZ
0388 603052

Darlington College
Cleveland Avenue
Darlington DL3 7BB
0325 467651

Derwentside College
Park Royal
Consett DH8 5EE
0207 502906

New College Durham
Framwell Moor Centre
Durham DH1 5ES
091-386 2421

Peterlee College
Burnhope Way
Peterlee 5R8 1NU
091-586 2225

Essex
Barking College
Dagenham Road
Romford RM7 0XU
0708 766841

Colchester Institute
Sheepen Road
Colchester CO3 3LL
0206 570271

Havering College
Ardleigh Green Road
Hornchurch RM11 2LL
04024 55011

Redbridge College
Little Heath
Romford RM6 4XT
081-599 5231

Thurrock College
Woodview
Grays RM16 4YR
0375 371621

Gloucestershire
Gloscat
Brunswick Road
Gloucester GL1 1HU
0452 426634

Royal Forest of Dean College
Berry Hill
Coleford GL16 7JT
0594 833416

Stroud College
Stratford Road
Stroud GL5 4AH
0453 763424

Greater Manchester
Bolton College
Manchester Road
Bolton BL2 1ER
0204 31411

Bury College
Market Street
Bury BL9 0BG
061-761 4327

Hopwood College
St Mary's Gate
Rochdale OL12 6RY
0706 345346

Oldham College
Rochdale Road
Oldham OL9 6AA
061-624 5214

Salford College
Walkden Road
Worsley
Manchester M28 4QD
061-702 8272

South Manchester College
Abraham Moss Centre
Crescent Road
Manchester M8 6UF
061-740 1491

Tameside College
Union Street
Hyde SK14 1ND
061-330 6911

Hampshire
Basingstoke College
Worting Road
Basingstoke RT21 1TN
0256 54141

Fareham Tertiary College
Bishopsfield Road
Fareham PO14 1NH
0329 220844

Farnborough College
Boundary Road
Farnborough GU14 6SB
0252 515511

Portsmouth College
Winston Churchill Avenue
Portsmouth PO1 2DJ
0705 826435

South Downs College
College Road, Purbrook Way
Havant PO7 8AA
0705 257011

Southampton College
St Mary Street
Southampton SO9 4WX
0703 635222

Herefordshire
Herefordshire College
Folly Lane
Hereford HR1 1LS
0432 267311

Hertfordshire
Hertford Regional College
Scotts Road
Ware SG12 9JF
0920 465441

Stevenage College
Monkswood Way
Stevenage SG1 1LA
0438 312882

West Herts College
Langley Road
Watford WD1 3RH
0923 240311

Humberside
East Yorks College
St Mary's Walk
Bridlington YO16 5JW
0262 672676

Grimsby College
Nuns Corner
Grimsby DN34 5BQ
0472 79292

Hull College
Queen's Gardens
Hull HU1 3DG
0482 29943

North Lindsey College
Kingsway
Scunthorpe DN17 1AJ
0742 281111

Ireland (Northern)
Ballymena College
Trostan Avenue
Ballymena
Co Antrim BT43 7BN
0266 652871

Belfast Institute
Tower Street
Belfast BT5 4FH
0232 452111

College of Further Education
400 Shore Road
Newtownabbey
Co Antrim BT37 9RS
0231 864331

Down College
Market Street, Downpatrick
Co Down
BT30 6ND
0396 615815

Dungannon College
Circular College
Co Tyrone BT71 6BQ
0868 722323

Fermanagh College
Enniskillen
Co Fermanagh BT47 6AE
0365 322431

Limavady College
Main Street, Limavady
Co Londonderry BT49 0EX
05047 62334

Lurgan College
Kitchen Hill, Lurgan
Co Armagh BT66 6AZ
0762 326135

Newry College
Patrick Street, Newry
Co Down BT35 8DN
0693 61071

North Down College
Victoria Avenue
Newtownards
Co Down BT23 3ED
0247 812116

North West College
Strand Road
Londonderry BT48 7BY
0504 266711

Isle of Man
Isle of Man College
Homefield Road
Douglas
0624 623113

Isle of Wight
Isle of Wight College
Medina Way
Newport PO30 5TA
0983 526631

Kent
Bromley College
Rookery Lane
Bromley BR2 8HE
081-462 6331

Erith College
Tower Road
Belvedere DA8 1PJ
03224 42331

Mid-Kent College
City Way
Rochester ME1 2AD
0634 830644

North West Kent College
Miskin Road
Dartford DA1 2LU
0322 225471

South Kent College
The Grange, Shorncliffe Road
Folkestone CT20 2NA
0303 850061

Thanet College
Ramsgate Road
Broadstairs CT10 1PN
0843 865111

West Kent College
Brook Street
Tonbridge TN9 2PW
0732 358101

Lancashire
Accrington and Rossendale
College
Rossendale Centre
Haslingden Road, Rawtenstall
BE4 6RA
0706 213558

Blackburn College
Feilden Street
Blackburn BB2 1LH
0254 55144

Blackpool and The Fylde College
Church Road
Lytham St Annes FY8 4AP
0252 52352

Lancaster and Morecambe
College
Morecambe Road
Lancaster LA1 2TY
0524 66215

Nelson and Colne College
Scotland Road
Nelson BB9 7YT
0282 603151

Oldham College
Rochdale Road
Oldham OL9 6AA
061-624 5214

Runshaw College
Langdale Road, Leyland, Preston
PR5 2DQ
0772 432511

Skelmersdale College
Yewdale Road
Skelmersdale WN8 6JA
0695 28744

Leicestershire
Coalville College
Bridge Road
Coalville LE6 2QR
0533 836136

Hinckley College
London Road
Hinckley LE10 1HQ
0455 251222

Melton Mowbray College
Asfordby Road
Melton Mowbray LE13 0HJ
0664 67431

South Fields College
Aylestone Road
Leicester LE2 7LW
0533 541818

Lincolnshire
Boston College
Rowley Road
Boston PE21 6JF
0205 365701

Grantham College
Stonebridge Road
Grantham NG31 9AP
0476 63141

Lincoln College
Lindum Road
Lincoln LN2 1NP
0522 23268

Stamford College
Drift Road
Stamford PE9 1XA
0780 64141

London Area
College of North East London
High Road
London N15 4RU
081-802 3111

Enfield College
Montague Building
73 Hertford Road
Enfield EN3 5HA
081-443 3434

Greenhill College
Lowlands Road
Harrow
Middlesex HA1 3AQ
081-422 2388

Hendon College
Corner Mead
Grahame Park
London NW9 5RA
081-200 8300

Hounslow Borough College
London Road
Isleworth, Middlesex TW7 4HS
081-568 0224/8

London College of Fashion
20 John Prince's Street
London W1M 9HG
071-629 9401

Newham Community College
West Ham Centre
Welfare Road, Stratford
London E15 4HT
081-472 1480

Tower Hamlets College
Clark Street
London E1 3HA
071-790 1066

Uxbridge College
Central Avenue
Hayes
Middlesex UB3 2DD
081-756 0414

Waltham Forest College
Forest Road
London E17 4JB
081-527 2311

Merseyside
City College
Colquitt Street
Liverpool L1 4DB
051-709 0541

Hugh Baird College
Balliol Road
Bootle L20 7EW
051-922 4040

St Helen's College
Brook Street
St Helens WA10 1PZ
0744 33766

Southport College
Mornington Road
Southport PR9 0TT
0704 42411

Wirral Metropolitan College
Carlett Park
Eastham, Wirral L62 0AY
051-327 4331

Norfolk
Great Yarmouth College
Southtown
Great Yarmouth NR31 0ED
0493 655261

Norfolk College
Tennyson Avenue
Kings Lynn PE30 2QW
0553 761144

Norwich City College
Ipswich Road
Norwich NR2 2LJ
0603 660011

Northamptonshire
Northampton College
Booth Lane South
Northampton NN3 3RF
0604 403322

Tresham College
George Street
Corby NN17 1QD
0536 203252

Nottinghamshire
Basford Hall College
Duke Street
Hucknall NG6 0ND
0602 637316

Clarendon College
Pelham Avenue
Mansfield Road, Nottingham
NG5 1AL
0602 607201

Newark and Sherwood College
Chauntry Park
Newark NG2 1PB
0636 705921

West Nottinghamshire College
Derby Road
Mansfield NG18 5BH
0623 27191

Oxfordshire
Henley College
Deanfield Avenue
Henley-on-Thames RG9 1UH
0491 573501

North Oxfordshire College
Broughton Road
Banbury OX16 9QA
0295 252221

Oxford College
Oxpens Road
Oxford OX1 1SA
0865 245871

Shropshire
Oswestry College
College Road
Oswestry SY11 2SA
0691 653067

Shrewsbury College
London Road
Shrewsbury SY2 6PR
0743 51544

Telford College
Haybridge Road
Wellington TF1 2NP
0952 641122

Somerset
Somerset College
Wellington Road
Taunton TA1 5AX
0823 283403

Strode College
Church Road
Street BA16 0AB
0458 42277

Yeovil College
Ilchester Road
Yeovil BA21 3BA
0935 23921

Staffordshire
Burton upon Trent College
Station Road
Stafford DE13 9AE
0283 520531

Cannock Chase College
Stafford Road
Cannock WS11 1VE
0543 462200

Newcastle-under-Lyme College
Liverpool Road
Newcastle ST5 2DF
0782 611531

Tamworth College
Croft Street
Tamworth B79 8AE
0827 310202

Suffolk
Suffolk College
Rope Walk, Ipswich IP4 1LT
0473 255885

West Suffolk College
Out Risbygate
Bury St Edmunds IP33 3AL
0284 701301

Surrey
Carshalton College
Nightingale Road
Carshalton SM5 2EJ
081-647 0021

Croydon College
The Crescent
Croydon CR9 2LY
081-684 9266

East Surrey College
Gatton Point
Redhill RH1 2FA
0737 766909

Guildford College
Stoke Park
Guildford GU1 1EZ
0483 31251

Kingston College
Kingston Hall Road
Kingston upon Thames KT1 2AQ
081-546 2151

Sussex
Brighton College
Pelham Street
Brighton BN1 4FA
0273 685971

Chichester College
Westgate Fields
Chichester PO19 1SB
0243 786321

Crawley College
College Road
Crawley RH10 1NR
0293 612686

Eastbourne College
Kings Drive
Eastbourne BN21 2HS
0323 644711

Hastings College
Archery Road
St Leonards-on-Sea TN38 0HX
0424 423847

Lewes College
Mountfield Road
Lewes BN7 7XH
0293 476121

Northbrook College
Broadwater Road
Worthing BN14 8HJ
0903 31445

Tyne and Wear
Gateshead College
Durham Road
Gateshead NE9 5BN
091-477 0524

Newcastle College
Sandyford Road
Newcastle NE1 8QE
091-232 6002

North Tyneside College
Embleton Avenue
Wallsend NE28 9NL
091-262 4081

South Tyneside College
St George's Avenue
South Shields NE34 6ET
091-456 0403

Wales
Afan College
Beechwood Road
Margam
Port Talbot
West Glamorgan SA13 2AL
0639 882107

Barry College
Colcot Road, Barry
South Glamorgan CF6 8YJ
0446 739593

Cardiff Institute
Colchester Avenue
Cardiff CF3 7XR
0222 151111

Carmarthenshire College
Alban Road
Llanelli
Dyfed SA15 1NG
0554 759165

Coleg Meiron Dwyfor
Barmouth Road
Dolgellau, Gwynedd LL40 2SW
0341 422827

Crosskeys College
Risca Road
Crosskeys, Gwent NP1 7ZA
0495 270295

Gwent Tertiary College
Nash Road
Newport, Gwent NP9 0TS
0633 274861

Gwynedd College
Friddoedd Road
Bangor, Gwynedd LL57 2TP
0248 364186

Llandrillo College
Llandudno Road, Rhos-on-Sea
Colwyn Bay, Clwyd LL28 4HZ
0492 546666

Montgomery College
Llanidloes Road
Newtown, Gwent SY16 4HU
0686 27444

North East Wales Institute
Kelston Lane
The Coach House
Connah's Bay
Clwyd CH5 4BR
0244 831531

Pembrokeshire College
Haverfordwest SA61 1SZ
0437 765247

Pontypool College
Blaendare Road
Pontypool, Gwent NP4 5YE
049 55 55141

Pontypridd College
Ynys Terrace, Rhydyfelin
Pontypridd, Mid Glamorgan
CF37 5RN
0443 400120

Rhondda College
Llwynypia, Tonypandy
Rhondda, Mid Glamorgan
CF40 2TQ
0443 432187

Rumney College
Trowbridge Road
Rumney
Cardiff CF3 8XZ
0222 794226

Warwickshire
Mid-Warwickshire College
Warwick New Road
Leamington Spa CV32 5JE
0926 311711

North Warwickshire College
Hinckley Road
Nuneaton CV11 6BH
0203 349321

West Midlands
Bilston College
Westfield Road
Bilston WV14 6ER
0902 353877

Birmingham College
Summer Row
Birmingham B3 1JB
021-235 3689

Coventry College
Butts
Coventry CV1 3GD
0203 257221

Dudley College
The Broadway
Dudley DY1 4AS
0384 455433

Hall Green College
Cole Bank Road
Birmingham B28 8ES
021-778 2311

Handsworth College
Soho Road
Handsworth, Birmingham
B21 9DP
021-551 6031

Sandwell College
Lodge Road
West Bromwich B70 8DW
021-556 6000

Solihull College
Blossomfield Road
Solihull B91 1SB
021-711 1719

Walsall College
St Paul's Street
Walsall WS1 1XN
0922 720824

Wiltshire
Chippenham College
Cocklebury Road
Chippenham SN15 3QD
0249 650501

Salisbury College
Southampton Road
Salisbury SP1 2PP
0722 26122

Swindon College
North Star Avenue
Swindon SN2 1DY
0793 491591

Trowbridge College
College Road
Trowbridge BA14 0ES
0225 766241

Worcestershire
Evesham College
Cheltenham Road
Evesham WR11 6LP
0386 41091

Kidderminster College
Hoo Road
Kidderminster DY10 1LX
0562 820811

North East Worcestershire
College
Peakman Street
Redditch B98 8DW
0527 63607

Worcester College
Deansway
Worcester WR1 2JF
0905 28383

Yorkshire
Barnsley College
Church Street
Barnsley S70 2AN
0226 299191

Bradford and Ilkley College
Great Horton Road
Bradford BD7 1AY
0274 753031

Calderdale College
Francis Street
Halifax HX1 3UZ
0422 358221

Castle College
Granville Road
Sheffield S2 2RL
0742 760271

Craven College
High Street
Skipton BD23 1JY
0756 791411

Doncaster Institute
Waterdale
Doncaster DN1 3EX
0302 322122

Harrogate College
Hornbeam Park, Hookstone Road
Harrogate HG9 8OT
0423 879466

Huddersfield College
New North Road
Huddersfield HD1 5NN
0484 536521

Keighley College
Cavendish Street
Keighley BD21 3DT
0535 618555

Rother Valley College
Doe Quarry Lane
Dinnington, Sheffield S31 7NH
0909 568681

Rotherham College
Eastwood Lane, Rotherham
S65 1EG
0709 362111

Selby College
Abbot's Road
Selby YO8 8AT
0757 702606

Shipley College
Exhibition Road
Shipley BD18 3JW
0274 595731

Thomas Danby College
Roundhay Road, Sheepscar
Leeds LS7 3BG
0532 494912

Wakefield District College
Whitwood Centre,
Four Lane Ends
Castleford WF10 5NF
0977 554571

York College
Dringhouses
York YO2 1UA
0904 704141

Yorkshire Coast College
Lady Edith's Drive, Scalby Road
Scarborough YO12 5RN
0723 372105

Private Establishments
and YT Centres
Alan Paul Training School
48 Great Charlotte Street
Liverpool L1 1PU
051-709 3165

Arndale House IPC
Cornhill, off Broadway
Accrington, Lancashire BB5 1EX
0254 398729

Park School of Beauty Therapy
Storcroft House, London Road
Retford, Nottinghamshire
DN22 7EB
0777 707371

Graham Austin Hair Design
222 Stamford Street
Ashton-under-Lyne, Lancashire
OL6 7LT
061-343 1159

Just-A-Head
101 Commercial Road
Portsmouth, Hampshire
PO1 1BQ
0705 295000

Michael John Training
228 Moss Lane
Bramhall, Stockport
Cheshire SK7 1BD
061-439 7029

Michol M (AWH) Ltd
2A High Street
Rotherham S60 1PP
0709 374445

Moorland Esthetiques
PO Box 491, Cheadle,
Greater Manchester ST10 2QL
0538 266771

Mr Constantine Hair Stylist
476-478 Broadway, Chadderton
Oldham, Lancashire OL9 9NS
061-682 7338

North Wales Youth Training
Agency
Mochdre Industrial Estate
Colwyn Bay, Clwyd LL28 5HE
0492 43431

South West Regional Productivity
Association
11 Basset Street
Camborne, Cornwall TR14 8SE
0209 710456

South West Regional Productivity
Association
3 Goldcroft
Yeovil, Somerset BA21 4DQ
0935 22726

J R Taylor (Fashions) Ltd
St Anne's on Sea
Lancashire FY8 2AB
0253 722266

West of England College
The Manor
Brewery Lane, Holcombe
Bath BA3 5EG
0761 232757

Ynys Mon, Isle of Anglesey
Training Centre
Industrial Estate, Llangefni
Anglesey LL77 7JA
0248 724760

Scottish Vocational Education Council (SCOTVEC)

Hanover House, 24 Douglas Street, Glasgow G2 7NQ; 041-248 7900

In Scotland, the Scottish Vocational Qualification (SVQ) is accredited by SCOTVEC and awarded by them and the Hairdressing Training Board.

Colleges offering hairdressing courses are:

Aberdeen College
Gallowgate
Aberdeen AB9 1DN
0224 640366

Banff and Buchan College
Argyll Road, Fraserburgh
Aberdeenshire AB4 5RF
0346 25777

Borders College
Thorniedean, Melrose Road
Galashiels TD1 2AF
0896 57755

Cambuslang College
Hamilton Road
Cambuslang G72 7NY
041-641 6600

Central College
300 Cathedral Street
Glasgow G1 2TA
041-552 3941

Clackmannan College
Branshill Road
Alloa FK10 3BT
02592 215121

Clydebank College
Kilbowie Road, Clydebank
Dumbartonshire G81 2AA
041-952 7771

Coatbridge College
Kildonan Street
Coatbridge ML5 3LS
0236 22316

Dumfries & Galloway College
Heathhall
Dumfries DG1 3QZ
0387 61261

Dundee College
Old Glamis Road
Dundee DD3 8LE
0382 819021

Esk Valley College
Newbattle Road, Eskbank
Dalkeith EH22 3AE
031-663 1951

Fife College
St Brycedale Avenue
Kirkcaldy KY1 1EX
0592 268591

Inverness College
Longman Road
Inverness IV1 1SA
0463 236681

James Watt College
Finnart Street
Greenock PA16 8HF
0475 24433

Kilmarnock College
Holehouse Road
Kilmarnock KA3 7AT
0563 23501

Moray College
Hay Street, Elgin IV30 2NN
0343 543425

Perth College
Crieff Road
Perth PH1 2NX
0738 21171

Telford College
Crewe Toll
Edinburgh EH4 2NZ
031-332 2491

Thurso College
Ormlie Road
Thurso
Caithness KW14 7EE
0847 66161

West Lothian College
Marjoribanks Street
Bathgate
West Lothian EH48 1QJ
0506 634300

Trichology

Institute of Trichologists (Incorporated)
228 Stockwell Road, London SW9 9SU; 071-733 2056

Colleges offering courses in trichology include:

Belfast Institute, Tower Street, Belfast BT5 4FH

City of Liverpool Community College, Colquitt Street, Liverpool L1 4DB

Clydebank College, Kilbowie Road, Clydebank G81 2AA

Huddersfield College, New North Road, Huddersfield HD1 5NN

Other colleges provide study by means of 'open learning' or 'flexistudy'.

Beauty

City and Guilds of London Institute
46 Britannia Street, London WC1X 9RG; 071-278 2468

The City and Guilds Beauty Therapy (304) scheme offers the full range of beauty treatments practised in beauty salons, health farms or health clinics. It covers manicure, pedicure, make-up, eyebrow and eyelash treatments, body and facial massage, removal of superfluous hair and exercise. Entry requirements are a minimum of three GCSEs (A–C) including English and a science; many colleges require higher qualifications.

Specialisms include Cosmetic Make-Up (302), Manicure (303) and Electrical Epilation (305).

Courses are offered at the following colleges:

Avon
Weston-super-Mare College
Knightstone Road
Weston-super-Mare BS23 2AL
0934 621301

Buckinghamshire
Aylesbury College
Oxford Road, Aylesbury
HP21 8PD
0296 434111

Cambridgeshire
Peterborough College
Park Crescent
Peterborough PE1 4DZ
0733 67366

Cheshire
South Cheshire College
Dane Bank Avenue
Crewe CW2 8AB
0270 69133

South Trafford College
Manchester Road
West Timperley
Altrincham WA14 5PQ
061-973 7064

Cleveland
Hartlepool College
Stockton Street
Hartlepool TS24 7NT
0429 275453

Kirby College
Roman Road, Middlesbrough
TS5 5PJ
0642 813706

Derbyshire
Chesterfield College
Infirmary Road, Chesterfield
S41 7NG
0246 231212

Derby College
Greenwich Drive South
Mackworth DE3 4FW
0332 518871

Devon
Exeter College
Hele Road, Exeter EX4 4JS
0392 273071

Plymouth College
Keppel Place
Stoke
Plymouth PL2 1AX
0752 382000

Dorset
Bournemouth and Poole College
Lansdowne, Bournemouth
BH1 3JJ
0202 295511

Durham
Darlington College
Cleveland Avenue, Darlington
DL3 7BB
0325 467651

Essex
Havering College
Ardleigh Green Road,
Hornchurch RM11 2LL
04024 55011

Thurrock College
Woodview, Grays RM16 4YR
0375 371621

Gloucestershire
Gloscat
Brunswick Road, Gloucester
GL1 1HU
0452 426504

Greater Manchester
Leigh College
Railway Road, Leigh WN7 4HX
0942 608811

Stockport College
Wellington Road, Stockport
SK1 3UQ
061-480 7331

Hertfordshire
Hertford Regional College
Scotts Road, Ware SG12 9JF
0920 465441

Humberside
Hull College
Queen's Gardens, Hull HU1 3DG
0482 29943

North Lindsey College
Kingsway, Scunthorpe DN17 1AJ
0742 281111

Isle of Man
Isle of Man College
Homefield Road
Douglas
0624 623113

Kent
Erith College
Tower Road, Belvedere, DA8 1PJ
03224 42331

Thanet College
Ramsgate Road, Broadstairs,
CT10 1PN
0843 865111

West Kent College
Brook Street, Tonbridge
TN9 2PW
0732 358101

Lancashire
Accrington and Rossendale
College
Rossendale Centre
Haslingden Road,
Rawtenstall BE4 6RA
0706 213558

Bolton College
Manchester Road
Bolton BL2 1ER
0204 31411

Lancaster and Morecambe
College
Morecambe Road
Lancaster LA1 2TY
0524 66215

Oldham College
Rochdale Road
Oldham OL9 6AA
061-624 5214

Preston College
St Vincents Road
Fulwood
Preston PR2 4UR
0772 716511

Leicestershire
South Fields College
Aylestone Road, Leicester
LE2 7LW
0533 541818

Lincolnshire
Boston College
Rowley Road
Boston PE21 6JF
0205 365701

Lincoln College
Lindum Road, Lincoln LN2 1NP
0522 522252

Stamford College
Drift Road
Stamford
PE9 1XA
0780 64141

London
College of North East London
High Road
London N15
071-802 3111

Hounslow Borough College
London Road, Isleworth
Middlesex TW7 4HS
081-568 0244/8

Newham College
Welfare Road
London E15 4HT
081-534 3958

Merseyside
Hugh Baird College
Balliol Road
Bootle
Liverpool L20 7EW
051-922 4040

St Helens College
Water Street, St Helens
WA10 1PZ
0744 33766

Wirral Metropolitan College
Carlett Park, Eastham
Wirral L62 0AY
051-327 4331

Northern Ireland
Ballymena College
Farm Lodge Avenue
Ballymena
Co Antrim BT43 7DJ
0266 652871

Belfast Institute
Tower Street
Belfast BT5 4FH
0232 452111

Rupert Stanley College
Tower Street, Belfast BT5 4FH
0232 52111

Norfolk
Norfolk College
Tennyson Avenue, Kings Lynn
PE30 2QW
0553 761144

Northamptonshire
Northampton College
Booth Lane South
Northampton NN3 3RF
0604 403322

Tresham College
George Street, Corby NN17 1QD
0536 203252

Nottinghamshire
Clarendon College
Pelham Avenue
Mansfield Road, Nottingham
NG5 1AL
0602 607201

Shropshire
Telford College
Haybridge Road
Wellington TF1 2NP
0952 641122

Somerset
Somerset College
Wellington Road
Taunton TA1 5AX
0823 283403

Strode College, Church Road
Street BA16 0AB
0458 42277

Staffordshire
Cannock Chase College
Stafford Road, Cannock
WS11 1VE
0543 462200

Suffolk
Lowestoft College
St Peter's Street
Lowestoft NR32 2WB
0502 583521

West Suffolk College
Out Risbygate, Bury St Edmunds
IP33 3RL
0284 701301

Surrey
Carshalton College
Nightingale Road
Carshalton 8MJ 2EJ
081-647 0021

Croydon College
The Crescent
Croydon CR0 2LY
081-684 9266

Guildford College
Stoke Park
Guildford EU1 1EZ
0483 31251

Kingston College
Kingston Hall Road
Kingston-upon-Thames KT1 2AQ
081-546 2151

Sussex
Brighton College
Pelham Street, Brighton
BN1 4FA
0273 685971

Chichester College
Westgate Fields, Chichester
PO19 1SB
0243 786321

Hastings College
Archery Road
St Leonards-on-Sea TN38 0HX
0424 423847

Tyne and Wear
Newcastle upon Tyne College
Maple Terrace
Newcastle upon Tyne NE4 7SA
091-273 8866

North Tyneside College
Embleton Avenue, Wallsend
NE28 9NL
091-262 4081

South Tyneside College
St George's Avenue
South Shields NE34 6ET
091-456 0403

Wales
Afan College
Beechwood Road, Margam
Port Talbot, West Glamorgan
SA13 2AL
0639 882107

Gwynedd College
Friddoedd Road, Bangor
Gwynedd LL57 2TP
0248 364186

Llandrillo College
Llandudno Road, Rhos-on-Sea
Colwyn Bay, Clwyd LL28 4HZ
0492 546666

Pontypridd College
Ynys Terrace, Rhydyfelin
Pontypridd, Mid Glamorgan
CF37 5RN
0443 400120

Warwickshire
Mid Warwickshire College
Warwick New Road
Leamington Spa CV32 5JE
0926 311711

North Warwickshire College
Hinckley Road, Nuneaton
CV11 6BH
0203 349321

West Midlands
Bilston College
Westfield Road, Bilston
WV14 6ER
0902 353877

Birmingham College
Summer Row, Birmingham
B3 1JB
021-235 2775

Dudley College
The Broadway
West Midlands DY1 4AS
0384 455433

Solihull College
Blossomfield Road, Solihull
B91 1SB
021-705 6376

Wiltshire
Swindon College
North Star, Swindon SN2 1DY
0793 491591

Trowbridge College
College Road, Trowbridge
BA14 0ES
0225 766241

Worcestershire
North East Worcestershire
College
Peakman Street, Redditch
B98 8DW
0527 63607

Yorkshire
Barnsley College
Church Street, Barnsley S70 2AN
0226 299191

Bradford and Ilkley College
Great Horton Road, Bradford
BD7 1AY
0274 753031

Calderdale College
Francis Street
Halifax HX1 3UZ
0422 358221

Castle College
Granville Road, Sheffield S2 2RL
0742 760271

Doncaster Institute
Waterdale, Doncaster DN1 3EX
0302 322122

Huddersfield College
New North Road, Huddersfield
HD1 5NN
0484 536521

Rotherham College
Eastwood Lane
Rotherham S65 1EG
0709 362111

Yorkshire Coast College
Lady Edith's Drive
Scalby Road, Scarborough
YO12 5RN
0723 372105

Private Establishments
Mary Bolton School
1 Private Road
Sherwood
Nottingham
0602 621866

The Park School of Beauty
Therapy
Storcroft House, London Road
Retford, Nottinghamshire
DN22 7EB
0777 860377

West of England College
The Manor
Brewery Lane
Holcombe
Bath BA3 53G
0761 232757

Business & Technology Education Council (BTEC)
Central House, Upper Woburn Place, London WC1H 0HH;
071-388 3288

The following colleges offer BTEC National Diploma courses in Beauty
Therapy:

Accrington and Rossendale
College
The Rossendale Centre
Haslingden Road
Rawtenstall, Rossendale
Lancashire BB4 6RA
0706 213558

Birmingham College
Summer Row
Birmingham B3 1JB
021-235 2775

Blackburn College
Feilden Street
Blackburn
Lancashire BB2 1LH
0254 55144

Bradford and Ilkley College
Great Horton Road, Bradford
BD7 1AY
0274 753031

Brighton College
Pelham Street
Brighton BN1 4FA
0273 685971

Cambridge College
Newmarket Road
Cambridge CB1 2NA
0223 357545

Chesterfield College
Infirmary Road, Chesterfield
S41 7NG
0246 231212

Chichester College
Westgate Fields, Chichester
PO19 1SB
0243 786321

Clarendon College
Pelham Avenue
Mansfield Road
Nottinghamshire NG5 1AL
0602 607201

College of North East London
Tottenham Centre
High Road
London N15 4RU
081-802 3111

Craven College
High Street
Skipton
North Yorkshire BD23 1JY
0756 791411

Crawley College
College Road
Crawley
West Sussex RH10 1NR
0293 612686

Erith College
Tower Road, Belvedere DA8 1PJ
03224 42331

Gateshead College
Durham Road
Gateshead
Tyne and Wear NE9 5BN
091-477 0524

Gloucestershire College
Oxstalls Lane
Gloucester GL2 9HW
0242 532000

Guildford College
Stoke Park, Guildford
Surrey GU1 1EZ
0483 31251

Hartlepool College
Stockton Street
Hartlepool
Cleveland TS24 7NT
0429 75423

Hull College
Queen's Gardens
Hull HU1 3DG
0482 29943

Kingston College
Kingston Hall Road
Kingston-upon-Thames
Surrey KT1 4AQ
081-546 2151

Kirby College
Roman Road
Middlesbrough TS5 5PT
0642 813706

Llandrillo College
Llandrillo Road
Rhos-on-Sea
Colwyn Bay
Clwyd LL28 4HZ
0492 546666

Leigh College
Railway Road
Leigh, Lancashire WN7 4AH
0942 608811

London College of Fashion
20 John Prince's Street
London W1M 0BJ
071- 629 9401

Northampton College
Booth Lane South
Northampton NN3 3RF
0604 403322

North East Worcestershire
College
Peakman Street
Redditch B98 8DW
0527 572867

North Tyneside College
Embleton Avenue
Tyne and Wear NE28 9NL
091-262 4081

North Warwickshire College
Hinckley Road
Nuneaton CV11 6BH
0203 349321

Pontypridd College
Ynys Terrace
Rhydyfelin
Pontypridd
Mid Glamorgan CF37 5RN
0443 400120

St Helens College
Brook Street
St Helens
Merseyside WA10 1PZ
051-744 33766

Somerset College
Wellington Road
Taunton
Somerset TA1 5AX
0823 283403

South Cheshire College
Dane Bank Avenue
Crewe
Cheshire CW2 8AB
0270 69133

South Fields College
Aylestone Road
Leicester LE2 7LW
0533 541818

South Manchester College
Moor Road
Wythenshawe
Manchester M23 9BQ
061-902 0131

Stockport College
Wellington Road South
Stockport SK1 3UQ
061-480 7331

Stoke-on-Trent College
Stoke Road
Shelton
Stoke-on-Trent
Staffordshire ST4 2DG
0782 202561

Thanet College
Ramsgate Road, Broadstairs
Kent CT10 1PN
0843 865111

Thomas Danby College
Roundhay Road
Sheepscat
Leeds L57 3BG
0532 494912

Tresham College
George Street
Corby NN17 1QD
Northamptonshire
0536 203252

Wirral Metropolitan College
Carlett Park
Eastham
Wirral, Cheshire L62 0AY
051-327 4331

The BTEC Higher National Diploma is offered by the London College of Fashion, and by Chichester, South Manchester and Stoke-on-Trent Colleges.

CIDESCO
UK schools recognised by CIDESCO are as follows:

Bretlands Beauty Centre
Baden Powell Place
Langton Road
Tunbridge Wells, Kent IN4 8XD
0892 533161

Cambridge School of Beauty
Therapy
94 High Street
Sawston, Cambridge CB2 4HJ
0223 832228

Champneys College of Health &
Beauty
Tring, Hertfordshire HP23 6HY
04427 873326

Great Yarmouth College
Southtown, Great Yarmouth
NR31 0ED
0493 655261

Henlow Grange Health Farm
Henlow, Bedfordshire SG16 6DP
0462 811111

Joan Price's Face Place Beauty
School
33 Cadogan Street, Chelsea
London SW3 2PP
071-589 9062

London Institute of Beauty
Culture
36 Dean Street
London W1V 5AP
071-287 0474

Mary Reid School of Beauty
59 Frederick Street
Edinburgh EH2 1LH
031-225 3167

Saltash College
Church Road, Saltash PL12 4AE
0752 844777

Park School of Beauty Therapy
Storcroft House, London Road
Retford, Nottinghamshire
DN22 7EB
0777 860377

Plymouth College
Kings Road
Devonport, Plymouth PL15 5QG
0752 264733

Ray Cochrane Training Centre
118 Baker Street
London W1M 1LB
071-486 6291

Roberta Mechan College
338 Lisburn Road, Belfast
BT9 6GH
0232 664960

Steiner School of Beauty Therapy
66 Grosvenor Street
London W1X 0AX
071-493 1146

The Retford College
Crown House
58a Bridgegate
Retford DN22 7UZ
0777 707371

West of England College
The Manor
Brewery Lane, Holcombe, Bath
BA3 53G
0761 232757

The Yorkshire College of Beauty
Therapy
The Manor
Haworth Lane
Yeadon, Leeds LS19 7EM
0532 509507

Confederation of International Beauty Therapy and Cosmetology

The examining body of the professional organisation is the British Association of Beauty Therapy and Cosmetology, Secretariat, 34 Imperial Square, Cheltenham, Gloucestershire GL50 1QZ.

To be accepted on a course you need a minimum of three GCSEs (A–C) or equivalent, one of which must be English and a second in human biology or other science subject. Courses are either in colleges of further education or private schools and last between six months and a year. Information on current fees can be obtained from the Confederation by sending an sae.

Schools and colleges running courses leading to the Confederation's diplomas include:

Avon
West of England College of Beauty Therapy
 The Manor, Brewery Lane, Holcombe BA3 5EG; 0761 232757

Bedfordshire
Henlow Grange
 Bedford SG16 6DP; 0462 811111

Cambridgeshire
Cambridge School of Beauty Therapy
 94 High Street, Sawston; 0223 832228

Cornwall
Saltash College
 Church Road, Saltash PL12 4AE; 0752 844777

Derbyshire
Chesterfield College
 Infirmary Road, Chesterfield S41 7NG; 0246 231212
Derby College
 Prince Charles Avenue, Mackworth, Derby DE22 LR4; 0332 519951

East Midlands College of Beauty
  Abbots Hill Chambers, Gower Street, Derby DE1 1SD; 0332 368195

Devon
North Devon College
  Barnstaple EX31 2BQ; 0271 45291
Plymouth College
  Kings Road, Devonport, Plymouth PL1 5QG; 0752 385314

Dorset
The International Beauty Academy Ltd
  487–489 Christchurch Road, Boscombe, Bournemouth BH1 4AE;
  0202 393039
Studio Olympus
  45 Bargates, Christchurch BH23 1QD; 0202 473210

Essex
Rogene School of Beauty
  Rogene House, 2a Chadwick Road, Ilford IG1 1BX; 081-478 2728
Thurrock College
  Woodview, Grays RM16 4YR; 0375 391199

Gloucestershire
Gloucestershire College
  Brunswick Campus, Brunswick Road, Gloucester GL1 1HU;
  0452 426630

Greater Manchester
Martindale School of Aesthetics
  175 Moorside Road, Flixton, Manchester M31 3SJ; 061-748 1213
Tameside College
  Beaufort Road, Ashton-under-Lyne, Tameside OL6 6NX;
  061-330 6911

Hampshire
Farnborough College
  Boundary Road, Farnborough GU14 6SB; 0252 515511
Southampton College
  St Mary Street, Southampton SO9 4WX; 0703 635222

Hertfordshire
Champneys College of Health & Beauty
  Wigginton, Tring HP23 6HY; 0442 873326

Kent
Maureen Austin School of Beauty Therapy
  1–2 Walden Parade, Walden Road, Chislehurst BR7 5DW;
  081-467 7135
Bretlands Beauty Centre
  Baden-Powell Place, Langton Road, Tunbridge Wells TN4 8XD;
  0892 533161

Erith College
  Tower Road, Belvedere DA17 6JA; 03224 42331
South Kent College
  Shorncliffe Road, Folkestone CT20 2NA; 0303 850061

London
Ray Cochrane Beauty School
  118 Baker Street, London W1M 1LB; 071-486 6291
London Institute of Beauty Culture
  36 Dean Street, London W1V 5AP; 071-287 0474
Joan Price's Face Place
  33 Cadogan Street, Chelsea, London SW3 2PP; 071-589 9062
Steiner School of Beauty Therapy
  Steiner House, 66 Grosvenor Street, London W1X 0AX;
  071-493 1146

Norfolk
Great Yarmouth College
  Southtown, Great Yarmouth NR31 0ED; 0493 655261

Nottinghamshire
Mary Bolton School
  1 Private Road, Sherwood, Nottingham; 0602 621866
Clarendon College
  Pelham Avenue, Nottingham NG5 1AL; 0602 607201
Park School of Beauty Therapy
  Storcroft House, London Road, Retford DN22 7EB; 0777 860377

Surrey
Kingston College
  Kingston Hall Road, Kingston upon Thames KT1 2AQ;
  081-546 2151
Lamontes Beauty Academy & Clinic
  220 High Street, Guildford GU1 3JD; 0483 38633
Susanne Saville School of Beauty Therapy
  Townsend House, 45a Dowing Street, Farnham GU9 7PH;
  0252 725671

Warwickshire
Mid-Warwickshire College
  Warwick New Road, Leamington Spa CV32 5JE; 0926 311711

West Midlands
Solihull College
  Blossomfield Road, Solihull B91 1SB; 021-711 1719

Yorkshire
Barnsley College
  Church Street, Barnsley S70 2AX; 0226 730191

Yorkshire Coast College
  Lady Edith's Drive, Scalby Road, Scarborough YO12 5RN;
  0723 372105
The Yorkshire College of Beauty Therapy
  The Manor, Haworth Lane, Yeadon, Leeds LS19 7EM; 0532 453676
White Rose School of Beauty
  2nd Floor, Standard House, George Street, Huddersfield HD1 4AD;
  0484 510625

Ireland
Bronwyn Conroy Ltd
  40 Grafton Street, Dublin 2; 0001 778783
The Coogan-Bergin College of Beauty Therapy
  Glendenning House, 6 Wicklow Street, Dublin 2; 0001 794254
Cork College of Beauty Training
  Emmet House, 8 Cross Street, Cork; 010 353 275741
Crumlin College
  Crumlin Road, Dublin 2; 0001 540662
FAS Training Centre
  Monavalley, Tralee, Co Kerry; 066 26444
Foxhall Beauty College
  Foxhall, Newport, Co Tipperary; 010 353 61378092
The Galligan College of Beauty
  109–110 Grafton Street, Dublin 2; 0001 792725
The Galligan College of Beauty
  Ard Ri House, Lower Abbeygate Street, Galway; 091 65628
The Galligan College of Beauty
  123 O'Connell Street, Limerick; 010 353 61410628
Senior College
  Blackrock, Eblana Avenue, Dun Laoghaire; 800385/6/7
Tralee Beauty Therapy College
  24 Denny Street, Tralee, Co Kerry; 010 353 6626690
Anne Weekes Beauty Ltd
  75 Waterloo Road, Dublin 4; 0001 689231
Woodworth/Whelan Therapy College
  16 Academy Street, Cork; 010 353 272507

Northern Ireland
The Constance Lutton Beauty Centre
  35 Kilmore Road, Lurgan, Craigavon, Co Armagh, BT67 9BP;
  0762 322267

Scotland
Perth College
  Brahan Estate, Crieff Road, Perth PH1 2NX; 0738 21171
Radix College of Beauty Culture
  West Sanquhar Road, Ayr KA8 9HP; 0292 261408

The International Health and Beauty Council
109 Felpham Road, Felpham, West Sussex PO22 7PW

The International Health and Beauty Council which together with the International Institute of Sports Therapy and the International Institute of Health and Holistic Therapies forms the Vocational Training Charitable Trust, 46 Aldwick Road, Bognor Regis, West Sussex PO21 2PN is at present the major provider of beauty therapy examinations in UK colleges.

Those colleges already offering the IHBC qualifications are planning to adopt the NVQ system this year and will need to satisfy inspectors that they have adequate facilities to retain assessment centre status. Candidates are advised to contact the Trust for a fuller and more up-to-date list of colleges and the colleges themselves for information about courses.

Courses
Diploma in Aesthetics – 3 GCSEs (A–C)
First Aid Certificate (normally an additional qualification)
Beauty Specialist's Diploma – 3 GCSEs (A–C)
Beauty Consultant's Certificate – 2GCSEs (A–C)
Certificate in Epilation – 2 GCSEs (A–C)
Cosmetic Make-up Certificate – 2 GCSEs (A–C) or alternatives as for 'Manicure Certificate'
Diploma in Health and Beauty Therapy – 4 GCSEs (A–C)
Diploma in Electrology – 3 GCSEs (A–C)
Health and Fitness Teacher's Diploma – 3 GCSEs (A–C)
International Beauty Therapist's Diploma – 4 GCSEs (A–C)
Body Massage Certificate – 2 GCSEs (A–C); or can be currently employed in a sauna establishment, public baths or beauty salon
Body Massage Diploma – 3 GCSEs (A–C); or employment as for the Certificate
International Master's Diploma in Health and Beauty Therapy – 2 A levels or 5 GCSEs (A–C) or other acceptable qualifications
Manicure Certificate – 2 GCSEs (A–C); or the course can be taken in conjunction with a hairdressing course, or full-time employment in a hairdressing or beauty salon
Make-up and Manicure Certificate – as for Manicure Certificate
Ear Piercing Certificate (normally an additional qualification)
Pedicure Endorsement
Remedial Camouflage Diploma – a basic facial qualification
Beauty Receptionist's Certificate – 2 GCSEs (A–C), unless the course is taken in conjunction with a hairdressing or beauty course, or the student is employed in a hairdressing or beauty salon
Sauna Treatments Diploma – 3 GCSEs, or employment as for Body Massage Certificate

International Beauty Teacher's Diploma – contact colleges for entry requirements
Theatrical and Media Make-Up Diploma – as for the Manicure Certificate
Cosmetic Ray Treatment Certificate (normally an additional qualification)

Recognised colleges offering these courses are as follows:

Local Authority Colleges

Avon
Brunel College
Mary Carpenter House
Ashley Down Road
Bristol BS7 9BU
0272 241241

City of Bath College
Avon Street
Bath BA1 1UP
0225 312191

Weston-super-Mare College
Knightstone Road
Weston-super-Mare BS23 2AL
0934 621301

Bedfordshire
Bedford College (Mander)
Cauldwell Street
Bedford MK42 9AH
0234 345151

Berkshire
Reading College
Crescent Road
Reading RG1 4RQ
0734 583501

Buckinghamshire
Aylesbury College
Oxford Road
Aylesbury HP21 8PD
0296 434111

Milton Keynes College
Chaffron Way
Leadenhall West
Milton Keynes MK6 5LP
0908 668998

Cambridgeshire
Cambridge College
Newmarket Road
Cambridge CB5 8EG
0223 357545

Channel Islands
Highlands College
PO Box 1000
St Saviour
Jersey
0534 71800

Cheshire
Halton College
Kingsway
Widnes WA8 7QQ
051-423 1391

North Cheshire College
Warrington North Campus
Winwick Road
Warrington WA2 8QA
0925 814343

South Trafford College
Manchester Road
West Timperley
Altrincham WA14 5PR
061-973 7064

West Cheshire College
Grange Centre
Regent Street
Ellesmere Port
South Wirral L65 8EJ
051-356 2300

Cleveland
Hartlepool College
Stockton Street
Hartlepool TS24 1NT
0429 275453

Kirby College
Roman Road
Linthorpe
Middlesbrough TS5 5PJ
0642 813706

Clwyd
Llandrillo College
Llandudno Road
Rhos-on-Sea
Colwyn Bay LL28 4HZ
0492 546666

Cornwall
Cornwall College
(Falmouth Centre)
Killigrew Street
Falmouth TR11 3QS
0326 313326

St Austell College
Palace Road
St Austell PL25 4BW
0726 67911

Cumbria
Carlisle College
Victoria Place
Carlisle CA1 1HS
0228 24464

Derbyshire
Chesterfield College
Infirmary Road
Chesterfield S41 7NG
0246 231212

Devon
Exeter College
Hele Road
Exeter EX4 4JS
0392 273071

South Devon College
Newton Road
Torquay TQ2 5BY
0803 213242

Durham
Bishop Auckland College
Woodhouse Lane
Bishop Auckland DL14 6JZ
0388 603052

Darlington College
Cleveland Avenue
Darlington DL3 7BB
0325 467651

Derwentside College
Park Royal
Consett DH8 5EE
0207 502906

New College Durham
Framwellgate Moor Centre
Durham DH1 5ES
091-386 2421

Peterlee College
Beverley Way
Howletch
Peterlee SR8 1NU
091-586 2225

Dyfed
Pembrokeshire College
Haverfordwest SA61 1SZ
0437 765247

East Sussex
Brighton College
Pelham Street
Brighton BN1 4FA
0273 685971

Eastbourne College
Kings Drive
Eastbourne BN21 2HS
0323 644711

Hastings College
Archery Road
St Leonards on Sea TN38 0HX
0424 423847

Lewes College
Mountfield Road
Lewes BN7 2XH
0273 483188

Essex
Harlow College
College Square
The High
Harlow CM20 1LT
0279 441288

Redbridge College
Little Heath
Romford RM6 4XT
081-599 5231

Thurrock College
Woodview
Grays RM16 4YR
0375 391199

Gwent
Crosskeys College
Riska Road
Crosskeys NP1 7ZA
0495 270295

Pontypool College
Blaendare Road
Pontypool NP4 5YE
04955 55141

Gwynedd
Coleg Meirion Dwyfor
Barmouth Road
Dolgellau LL40 2SW
0341 422827

Gwynedd College
Ffriddoedd Road
Bangor LL57 2TP
0248 370125

Hampshire
Basingstoke College
Worting Road
Basingstoke RG12 1TN
0256 54141

Eastleigh College
Chestnut Avenue
Eastleigh SO5 5HT
0703 644011

Farnborough College
Boundary Road
Farnborough GU14 6SB
0252 515511

Portsmouth College
Winston Churchill Avenue
Portsmouth PO1 2DJ
0705 826435

South Downs College
College Road
Havant PO7 8AA
0705 257011

The Tertiary College Fareham
Bishopsfield Road
Fareham PO14 1NH
0329 220844

Hereford and Worcester
Kidderminster College
Hoo Road
Kidderminster DY10 1LX
0562 820811

North East Worcester College
School Drive
Stratford Road
Bromsgrove B60 1PQ
0527 79500

Worcester College
Deansway
Worcester WR1 2JF
0905 723383

Hertfordshire
West Herts College
Langley Road
Watford WD1 3RH
0923 240311

Isle of Man
Isle of Man College
Homefield Road
Douglas
0624 623113

Isle of Wight
Isle of Wight College
Medina Way
Newport PO30 5TA
0983 526631

Kent
Bromley College
Rookery Lane
Bromley
Kent BR2 8HE
081-462 6331

Erith College
Tower Road
Belvedere DA17 6JA
03224 42331

North West Kent College
Miskin Road
Dartford DA1 2LU
0322 225471

South Kent College
Shorncliffe Road
Folkestone CT20 2NA
0303 850061

Thanet College
Ramsgate Road
Broadstairs CT10 1PN
0843 865111

West Kent College
Brook Street
Tonbridge TN9 2PW
0732 358101

Lancashire
Accrington and Rossendale
College
The Rossendale Centre
Haslingden Road
Rawtenstall
Rossendale BB4 6RA
0706 213558

Blackburn College
Feilden Street
Blackburn BB2 1LH
0254 55144

Blackpool and Fylde College
Ansdall Site
Church Road
Lytham St Annes FY8 4AP
0253 293071

Bury Metropolitan College
Market Street
Bury BL9 0BG
061-763 1505

Lancaster and Morecambe
College
Morecambe Road
Lancaster LA1 2TY
0524 66215

Oldham College
Rochdale Road
Oldham OL9 6AA
061-624 5214

Leicestershire
South Fields College
Aylestone Road
Leicester LE2 7LW
0533 541818

Lincolnshire
Lincoln College
Lindum Road
Lincoln LN2 1NP
0522 522252

Stamford College
Drift Road
Stamford PE9 1XA
0780 64141

London
College of North East London
High Road
London N15 4RU
081-802 3111

Hendon College
Corner Mead
Grahame Park
London NW9 5RA
081-200 8300

Waltham Forest College
Forest Road
Walthamstow E17 4JB
081-527 2311

Manchester
Salford College
Worsley Campus
Walken Road
Worsley M28 4QD
061-702 8272

South Manchester College
Wythenshawe Park Centre
Moor Road
Wythenshawe M23 9BQ
061-998 5511

Merseyside
Hugh Baird College
Balliol Road
Bootle L20 7EW
051-922 4040

St Helens College
Brook Street
St Helens WA10 1PZ
0744 33766

Southport College
Mornington Road
Southport PR9 0TT
0704 500606

Wirral College
Carlett Park
Eastham
Wirral L62 0AY
051-327 4331

Mid Glamorgan
Pontypridd College
Ynys Terrace
Rhydyfelin CS37 5RN
0443 486121

Rhondda College
Llwynypia
Tonypandy CF40 2TQ
0443 432187

Norfolk
Norfolk College
Tennyson Avenue
Kings Lynn PE30 2QW
0553 761144

Northamptonshire
Northampton College
St Gregory's Road
Booth Lane South
Northampton NN3 3RF
0604 403322

Tresham College
Corby Centre
Corby NN17 1QA
0536 402252

Northern Ireland
Belfast Institute
Tower Street
Belfast BT5 4FH
0232 452111

North Down & Ards College
Park Road
Bangor
Co Down BT20 4TF
0247 271254

Oxfordshire
Oxford College
Oxpens Road
Oxford OX1 1SA
0865 245871

Powys
Coleg Powys
Spa Road
Llandrindod Wells LD1 5ES
0597 2696

Shropshire
Telford College
Haybridge Road
Wellington
Telford TF1 2NP
0952 641122

Somerset
Somerset College
Wellington Road
Taunton TA1 5AX
0823 283403

South Glamorgan
Barry College
Colcot Road
Barry CF62 8YJ
0446 739593

South Yorkshire
Sheffield College
Granville Road
Sheffield S2 2RL
0742 760271

Staffordshire
Burton-upon-Trent College
Station Road
Stafford DE13 9AE
0283 520531

Strathclyde
Clydebank College
Kilbowie Road
Clydebank G81 2AA
041-952 7771

Suffolk
West Suffolk College
Out Risbygate
Bury St Edmunds IP33 3RL
0284 701301

Surrey
East Surrey College
Gatton Point
Alpine Road
Redhill RH1 2FA
0737 766909

Tyne and Wear
Gateshead College
Durham Road
Gateshead NE9 5BN
091-477 0524

Newcastle College
Sandyford Road
Newcastle upon Tyne NE1 8QE
091-232 6002

North Tyneside College
Embleton Avenue
Willington Quay
Wallsend NE28 9NJ
091-262 4081

South Tyneside College
St George's Avenue
South Shields NE34 6ET
091-456 0403

Warwickshire
North Warwickshire College
Hinckley Road
Nuneaton CV11 6BH
0203 349321

West Glamorgan
Afan College
Beechwood Road
Margam
Port Talbot SA13 2AL
0639 882107

West Midlands
Bilston College
Westfield Road
Bilston WV14 6ER
0902 353877

Birmingham College
Summer Row
Birmingham B3 1JB
021-235 3689

Coventry College
The Butts
Coventry CV1 3GU
0203 257221

Dudley College
The Broadway
Dudley DY1 4AS
0384 455433

Handsworth College
The Council House
Soho Road
Handsworth B21 9DP
021-551 6031

Sandwell College
Wednesbury Campus
Woden Road South
Wednesbury WS10 0PE
021-556 6000

Walsall College
St Paul's Street
Walsall WS1 1XN
0922 720824

West Sussex
Crawley College
College Road
Crawley RH10 1NR
0293 612686

West Yorkshire
Thomas Danby College
Roundhay Road
Sheepscar
Leeds LS7 3BG
0532 494912

Wiltshire
Chippenham College
Cocklebury Road
Chippenham SN15 3QD
0249 650501

Swindon College, North Star
Avenue
Swindon SN2 1DY
0793 491591

Trowbridge College
College Road
Trowbridge BA14 0ES
0225 766241

Independent Centres (UK)
Anne Hammond College
70 Woodthorne Road South
Tettenhall
Wolverhampton WV6 8SL
0902 752308

Belbins House Health and Beauty
Academy
Belbins House
Romsey
Hampshire SO51 0PE
0794 512226

The Berkshire Academy
42 Bartholomew Street
Newbury
Berkshire
0635 43607

Biocraft Hair and Beauty
Training Centre
Unit 105
Jubilee Trades Centre
130 Pershore Street
Birmingham B5 6ND
021-622 4749

Bishop College of Beauty
Therapy
West Layton Manor
West Layton
Richmond
North Yorkshire DL11 7PP
0325 718688

Bryn-y-Mor House of Beauty
20 Bryn-y-Mor Road
Swansea
West Glamorgan SA1 4JJ
0792 468804

Burghley Academy of Beauty
19 Burghley Road
Peterborough
Cambridgeshire PE1 2QA
0733 47126

Claire Walsham School of Beauty
New Identity Hair and Beauty
Salon
1089 Chester Road
Erdington
Birmingham
021-373 7532

Henlow Grange College
Henlow Grange Health Farm
Henlow
Bedfordshire SG16 6DP
0462 811111

La Femme Health and Beauty
Clinic
37 London Road
Alderley Edge
Cheshire SK9 7JT
0625 585851

'Mala' Beauty School
9 Greenhill
Evesham
Worcestershire WR11 4LX
0386 49400

Martin James Hair and Beauty
Design Group
New Road Complex
New Road
Kidderminster
Worcestershire DY10 1HJ
0562 67980/745879

Quantum YTS
Thornton House
Cemetery Road
Shelton
Stoke on Trent
Staffordshire ST4 2DL
0782 202366

South West Regional Productivity
Association
Basset House
11 Basset Road
Camborne
Cornwall TR14 8SE
0209 710456

South West Regional Productivity
Association
Flemming House
3 Goldcroft
Yeovil
Somerset BA21 4DQ
0935 22726

Top to Toe College of Beauty
Therapy
Well Lane House
off High Street
Haslemere
Surrey GU27 2LB
0428 2965

West of England College of
Beauty Therapy and
Hairdressing
The Manor,
Brewery Lane
Holcombe
Bath
Avon BA3 5EG
0761 232757

The International Therapy Examination Council
James House, Oakelbrook Mill, Newent, Gloucestershire GL18 1HD; 0531 821875

ITEC is an independent body which provides a professional examination system covering all aspects of therapy and beauty. Courses leading to the certificates and diplomas of the Council are held either in colleges of further education or in private schools, and last on average between six months and a year. You must be 18 by the time you sit the examinations. Minimum educational requirement is five GCSEs (A-C) or equivalent, preferably including English language and biology.

Exam Subjects
Beauty Therapy: Covers beauty therapy, body massage, vacuum suction, faradism (the use of a passive muscle exerciser for slimming treatments), galvanism (a treatment for very dry or greasy facial skin, also used for slimming), high frequency (used for facial treatments) etc.
Aestheticienne: Covers beauty and make-up.
Physiatrics: Covers therapy, body massage, vacuum suction and faradism, galvanism etc.
Beauty Consultancy: Designed for students intending to work as cosmetic consultants.
Electrology
Manicure
Anatomy and Physiology
Anatomy, Physiology and Massage Diploma
Teacher Training
Clinical Camouflage Make-up
Sports Therapy
Reflexology
Aromatherapy
Facial Make-up
Special Professions
Stage and Character Make-up
Aerobics
Gym Instructors
Nutrition and Diet
Holistic Clinical Honours Diploma

Courses leading to ITEC examinations are offered at:

London
Academy of Beauty Culture
5 South Dene
Mill Hill
London NW7 3BE
081-959 6728

Avdji Academy of Beauty
97-99 Upper Street
London N1 2XQ
071-226 4970

The Boyesen Centre
Acacia House, Centre Avenue
The Vale, Acton Park
London W3 7JX
081-743 2437

The Churchill Centre
22 Montagu Street
London W1H 1TB
071-402 9475

Community Health Foundation
188–194 Old Street
London EC1V 9BD
071-251 4076

Denleigh School of Beauty
Therapy
12 Uxbridge Road
Hampton
Middlesex TW12 3AD
081-946 3898

Greenwood College of Health and
Beauty
176 Kensington High Street
London W8
071-937 6595

Hounslow Borough College
London Road, Isleworth
Middlesex TW7 4HS
081-568 0244

London Academy of Beauty
512 Alkham Road
Stoke Newington
London N16 7AA
081-806 2788

Morley College
61 Westminster Bridge Road
London SE1 7HT
071-928 8501

The Village Affair School of
Beauty Therapy
32–34 The Ridgeway
Wimbledon Village
London SW19 4QW
081-946 6222

Wendover House College of
Beauty Therapy
Wendover House
Beaconsfield Road
Friern Barnet, London N11 3AB
081-361 8161

Wendy Rigby School of Massage
3 Ellerdale Road
London NW3 6BA
071-435 5407

West London School of
Therapeutic Massage
41 St Luke's Road
London W11 1DD
071-299 4672

Southern England
Aylesbury College
Oxford Road, Aylesbury
Buckinghamshire HP21 8PD
0296 434111

Beaumont College of Natural
Medicine
16 Dittons Road
Eastbourne BN21 1DW
0323 641676

Berkshire School of Natural
Therapy
Conifers
21 Dukes Wood
Crowthorne
Berkshire RG11 6NF
0344 761715

Bournemouth School of Massage
14 Greenwood Road
Bournemouth BH9 2LH
0202 513838

Bridgwater College
Bath Road
Bridgwater
Somerset TA16 4PZ
0278 455464

Cambridge School of Beauty
Therapy
94 High Street, Sawston
Cambridge CB2 4HJ
0223 832228

Cheltenham Therapy Training
Centre
2 Norwood House
6 Lansdowne Crescent
Cheltenham
Gloucestershire GL50 2JY
0242 224283

East Devon College
Department of Arts and Adult
Education
Bolham Road, Tiverton
Devon EX16 6SH
0884 254247

Essex School of Massage
Hadleigh Rise
Middle Street
Nazeing
Essex EN9 2LH
0992 892110

Gablecroft College of
Natural Therapy
Church Street, Whittington
Oswestry
Shropshire SY11 4DT
0691 659631

Health and Harmony School of
Beauty Therapy
19 West Street, Wilton
Wiltshire SP2 0DL
0722 743995

Henley College
Deanfield Avenue
Henley-on-Thames
Oxfordshire RG9 1UH
0491 579988

Langley College
Station Road, Langley
Slough, Berkshire SL3 8BY
0753 549222

Larosa School
17 Southdown Close
Brixham
Devon TQ 0AQ
08045 58571

Millfield School of Beauty
Millfield House, Rusper
Nr Horsham, Sussex
0293 871406

Raworth Centre for Natural
Health Studies
'Smallburgh', Beare Green
Dorking, Surrey RH5 4QA
0306 712623

Redbridge College
Little Heath, Romford
Essex RM6 4XT
081-599 5231

Rogene School of Beauty Therapy
Rogene House
2A Chadwick Road
Ilford, Essex IG1 1BX
081-478 2728

School of Physical Therapies
Lauriston
London Road
Basingstoke
Hampshire RG21 2AA
0256 475728

Solaire International College
of Beauty
Solaire House, Lucas Close
Yateley, Camberley
Surrey GU17 7JD
0252 873334

Stewart Michell Massage Practice
and Training
38 South Street
Exeter EX4 1ED
0392 410855

Strode College
Church Road
Street
Somerset BA16 0AB
0458 42277

Susanne Saville School of
Beauty Therapy
Townsend House,
45A Downing Street
Farnham, Surrey GU9 7PH
0252 725671

Threeways College
Yelverton Road
Framingham Earl
Norwich NR14 7SD
05086 3478

Trowbridge College
College Road
Trowbridge
Wiltshire BA14 0ES
0225 766241

West of England College of
Beauty Therapy
The Manor
Brewery Lane
Holcombe
Bath BA3 3PY
0761 232757

Wilbury Clinic of Natural
Medicine
64 Wilbury Road, Hove
Sussex BN3 3PY
0273 24420

Yeovil College
Ilchester Road
Yeovil
Somerset BA21 3BA
0935 23921

Northern England
Barnsley College
Church Street
Barnsley S70 2AX
0226 7301191

Clarendon College
515 Hagley Road
Birmingham B66 4AX
021-429 9191

East Yorkshire College
St Mary's Walk
Bridlington
East Yorkshire YO16 5JW
0262 672676

Gablecroft College of Natural
Therapy
Church Street
Whittington
Oswestry
Shropshire SY11 4DT
0691 659631

Lancashire Holistic College
65a Adelphi Street
Preston
Lancashire PR1 7BH
0772 25177

Leeds Central School of Beauty
8 King Charles Street
Leeds LS1 6LT
0532 434343

Nantwich School of Beauty
2 Marsh Lane, Nantwich
Cheshire CW5 5HH
0270 629619

Park School of Beauty Therapy
Storcroft House
London Road, Retford
Nottinghamshire DN22 7EB
0777 860377

The Retford College
58a Bridgegate
Retford
Nottinghamshire DN22 7UX
0777 707371

Sylvia Brearley Massage School
17 Rossett Holt Close
Harrogate HG2 9AD
0423 505707

West Herts College
Langley Road
Watford
Hertfordshire WD1 3RH
0923 240311

White Rose School of Beauty
Standard House
George Street
Huddersfield
W Yorkshire HD1 4AD
0484 510625

York College of Arts
and Technology
Dringhouses, York YO2 1UA
0904 704141

Yorkshire College of Beauty
Malmouth
Howorth's Lane
Yesdon
Yorkshire LS19 7EN
0532 509507

Scotland
Mary Reid School of
Beauty Culture
57 Patrick Street
Edinburgh EH2 1LH
031-225 3167

Radix College of Beauty Culture
West Sanquhar Road
Ayr KA8 9HP
0292 289374

Northern Ireland
Flamingo Health and Beauty
Ballymena Street
Ballymena, Co Antrim
0266 059598
(Aerobics only)

Roberta Mechan College of
Beauty
338 Lisburn Road
Belfast BT9 6GH
0232 664940

Wales
Butetown Community Centre
Loudoun Square
Butetown
Cardiff CF1 5JA
0222 487 6588

North Wales Clinic Of Relaxation
Roslyn
The Promenade
Llanfairfechan
Gwynedd LL33 0BY
0248 68706

For a full list contact ITEC at the above address.

Massage

Northern Institute of Massage
100 Waterloo Road, Blackpool FY4 1AW; 0253 403548

The Northern Institute offers two basic courses:

1. Body massage and physical culture.
2. Remedial massage.

The Institute conducts these courses by a mixture of correspondence tuition and practical study, most of the theoretical section of the training being studied at home. There are no educational requirements to enter a course, except that you should be 18 or over. All students are accepted on a one-month trial basis.

You obtain the required practical instruction for diploma qualification by means of attendance at short-period practical training sessions at appropriate stages of training.

A busy all-year-round programme of practical classes takes place at the Institute at Blackpool and occasionally in London, thus allowing the new student to commence the practical training of the basic courses when he or she is ready to do so, without having to wait for 'starting dates' of courses. Classes are arranged mainly at weekends for the convenience of students in full-time occupation. Also, mid-week classes are held at frequent intervals for the benefit of students who wish to cover as much practical instruction as possible on the occasion of a visit to the college.

The student may choose, therefore, to attend for practical instruction at Blackpool or, if more convenient, at weekend classes in London, supervised by tutors from or approved by the Institute.

The length of training can vary considerably with each individual student, but there is absolutely no time limit to any student's training. The student is permitted to proceed at his or her own pace and convenience throughout.

Remedial Massage Course
This course provides a thorough introduction to remedial massage theraphy for students who seek to work in health hydros and similar establishments, as assistants to practising therapists, with sports clubs, or in private practice.

The method of study and qualification in this course may be undertaken by a programme of home-study of 14 theoretical lessons, supplemented and linked to the necessary practical tuition periods (105 hours) at appropriate stages during the training.

The theoretical instruction of the course involves a study of anatomy and physiology at somewhat greater depth than in the Body Massage and Physical Culture Course, and the syllabus is extended to provide the student also with an understanding of the therapeutic benefits (and contra-indications) of massage in the treatment of certain conditions and injuries.

Advanced Study Group

The Advanced Study Group is a further educational service of the Northern Institute of Massage which keeps its members in constant contact with an established tuition organisation.

Through the Group, members may receive instruction in advanced remedial massage and allied subjects, such as electro-therapy etc, or in specialised techniques. Such instruction is provided by means of literature available to the member, and by attendance at practical classes, seminars etc.

Reflexology

The British School of Reflexology offers a four-part training course. Sessions are held mid-week and at weekends. Courses are held in Bristol, Harlow, Harrogate, London and Nottingham.

Attendance at the school on alternate months, together with a correspondence course, leads, over a period of at least eight months, to examinations for the school's diploma. Membership of the Holistic Association of Reflexologists is then offered which includes Membership of the British Complementary Medicine Association (BCMA).

Further information, including details of a book and charts, from: The British School of Reflexology, Holistic Healing Centre, 92 Old Sheering Road, Old Harlow, Essex CM17 0JW.

Reflexology courses are also offered by some of the International Therapy Examination Schools (see pp 86–90).

Electrolysis

Institute of Electrolysis

Lansdowne House, 251 Seymour Grove, Manchester M16 0DS; 061-881 5306

The Institute offers a full-time course of training, leading to the examination for the Diploma in Remedial Electrolysis. Those candidates eligible to sit for the diploma examination must satisfy the Council that:

(a) they have received a full-time course of training *either* in electrolysis to an approved standard, of at least 600 hours, including no less than 300 hours of practical work, *or*

(b) they have been in continuous practice for a period of at least two years.

There are no exemptions from any part of the diploma examinations (examinations are held annually, usually in London; dates can be obtained from the Secretary at the above address).

No specific educational qualifications are required, but you should have a good standard of education and some aptitude for the practical side of the work. GCSE English and human biology are helpful.

The syllabus covers anatomy and physiology; the endocrine system; detailed study of skin and hair; clinical pathology; electrolysis; practice organisation; patients; first aid. There is also a separate examination in sterilisation procedures, particularly important in view of the risks of AIDS and viral hepatitis.

The following is a list of registered tutors who should be contacted direct, but in writing rather than by telephone as they may be busy during normal clinic hours.

List of Registered Tutors
Barnt Green, Birmingham
Mrs I Clarke DRE, 38 Twatling Road, Birmingham B45 8MU; 021-445 2149

Bedford
Mrs K Treby DRE, Spinney Hill House, Sharnbrook, Souldrop MK44 1EX; 0234 781028

Deal, Kent
Ms M Jamieson DRE, Deal Electrolysis Beauty Clinic, 21 Lever Street; 0304 360656

Hotspur, Nr Beaconsfield, Buckinghamshire
Mrs J Jones DRE, 99 Heath Road, HP9 1DG

Maidstone, Kent
Mrs A J S Wheat DRE, 5 Hornbeam Close, Larkfield, ME20 61Y

Manchester
Mrs E Derbyshire DRE, Lansdowne House, 251 Seymour Grove, M16 0DS; 061-881 5306

Newcastle
Mrs Tonia Reed, Park Beauty Clinic, 142 Northumberland Street,
NE1 7DQ; 091-232 6682

Reading, Berkshire
Mrs N McGready DRE, 66 Erleigh Court Gardens, Earley; 0734 662828

Sheffield, Yorkshire
Mrs C A Clarke, 'Beauty by Christine Clarke', 428A Eccleshall Road,
S11 8PX; 0742 682140

West Worthing, Sussex
Mrs F Godfrey DRE, 2 Fulmer Court, Boundary Road, Worthing;
0903 202871

Chapter 8
Useful Addresses

The British Association of Beauty Therapy and Cosmetology Ltd
Secretariat, 34 Imperial Square, Cheltenham, Gloucestershire
GL50 1QZ

The British Association of Professional Hairdressing Employers
1A Barbon Close, Great Ormond Street, London WC1N 3JX

The British School of Reflexology, Holistic Healing Centre
92 Old Sheering Road, Old Harlow, Essex CM17 0JW

Business & Technology Education Council (BTEC)
Central House, Upper Woburn Place, London WC1 0HH

City and Guilds of London Institute
46 Britannia Street, London WC1X 9RG

Hairdressing Council
12 David House, 45 High Street, London SE25 6HJ

Hairdressing Training Board
3 Chequer Road, Doncaster DN1 2AA

Health and Beauty Therapy Training Board
PO Box 21, Bognor Regis, West Sussex PO 22 7PS

Institute of Electrolysis
Lansdowne House, 251 Seymour Grove, Manchester M16 0DS

Institute of Trichologists
228 Stockwell Road, London SW9 9SU

International Federation of Aromatherapists
Royal Masonic Hospital, Ravenscourt Park, London W6 0TN

International Health and Beauty Council
109 Felpham Road, Felpham, West Sussex PO22 7PW

International Therapy Examination Council
James House, Oakelbrook Mill, Newent, Gloucestershire GL18 1HD

National Council for Vocational Qualifications
222 Euston Road, London NW1 2EB

National Hairdressers Federation
11 Goldington Road, Bedford MK40 3JY

Northern Institute of Massage
100 Waterloo Road, Blackpool FY4 1AW

Scottish Vocational Education Council (SCOTVEC)
Hanover House, 24 Douglas Street, Glasgow G2 7NQ

Vocational Training Charitable Trust, incorporating the International
Health and Beauty Council, the International Institute of Sports
Therapy and the International Institute of Health and Holistic
Therapies
46 Aldwick Road, Bognor Regis, West Sussex PO21 2PN

Useful Journals

Hair
Southbank Publishing Group, King's Reach Tower, Stamford Street,
London SE1 9LS. Quarterly.

Hairdresser's Journal International
Reed Business Publishing Group, Quadrant House, The Quadrant,
Sutton, Surrey SM2 5AS. Weekly.

Health and Beauty Salon
Reed Business Publishing Group, address above. Monthly.

The National Hairdresser
Journal of the National Hairdressers Federation, 11 Goldington Road,
Bedford MK40 3JY. Bi-monthly.